The MRCPsych Study Manual

Third Edition

Edited by

Ben Green MRCPsych, ILTM
Consultant Psychiatrist and Clinical Tutor
Cheadle Royal Hospital
Honorary Senior Lecturer
University of Liverpool

Radcliffe Publishing
Oxford ● Seattle

Radcliffe Publishing Ltd
18 Marcham Road
Abingdon
Oxon OX14 1AA
United Kingdom

www.radcliffe-oxford.com
Electronic catalogue and worldwide online ordering facility.

First edition 1993 (published by Kluwer Academic Publishers)
Second edition 2000 (published by LibraPharm Ltd)

British Library Cataloguing in Publication Data

A catalogue record for this book is available from the British Library.

ISBN-10: 1 85775 684 3
ISBN-13: 978 1 85775 684 5

Typeset by Advance Typesetting Ltd, Oxford
Printed and bound by TJ International Ltd, Padstow, Cornwall

Contents

Preface to the third edition

It is unusual for an exam-related book to reach a second edition let alone a third, but I am pleased to say that previous editions of *The MRCPsych Study Manual* have met with good sales and reviews, hence the renewal of the book that represents this third edition.

Six years have elapsed since the last edition. Much has changed with regard to the MRCPsych examination and there has been a need to radically restructure the *Manual* and also a great proportion of the text is brand new. I am indebted to the new contributors. The text still contains some elements from previous editions and their contributors are acknowledged in these past volumes.

Please do write to me or email me if there are any comments or suggestions for improvements that you think should grace any future edition.

May potential candidates who use this book enjoy success.

Ben Green
January 2006
bengreen@liv.ac.uk

Preface to the second edition

This new edition of *The MRCPsych Study Manual* has given us a chance to update the old material, incorporate reviewers' and readers' comments and to add brand new sections. The result is an expanded and hopefully current edition with all-new chapters on essay writing, the Critical Review Paper, and a wholly new set of Multiple-Choice Questions (MCQs) for Part I.

Please do write to me or email me if there are any comments or suggestions for improvements that you think should grace any future edition.

I am indebted to my fellow contributors for their wisdom, timeliness, and good humour.

May potential candidates who use this book enjoy success.

Ben Green, 1999

Preface to the first edition

This book is not intended as a textbook. Nor is this book purely an examination aid. Its aim is to show the relevance of questions and subjects often addressed in the Membership of the Royal College of Psychiatrists (MRCPsych) examination. In showing the relevance of these questions and their relationship to current opinion we hope that candidates will gain a better understanding of the literature. Hopefully this will lead to a sense of how they can best organise their limited time for revision. Candidates can then gain as much enjoyment and knowledge as possible while they are preparing for their examinations. After all, the MRCPsych examination is not an end in itself; it is merely a symbol of a continuing educational process. We hope the book will stimulate the reader to work through its questions and through following up suggested references develop an expanding interest in the whole field of psychiatry. The ability to continually re-educate oneself will be a vital skill because continuing medical education will be a key feature in future European training.

The *Manual* covers both Part I and Part II of the MRCPsych examination, because the examinations are not discrete entities, but are parts of a training process.

The book should be used well before both exams. Suggestions for developing a study programme are given in the first section. The best self-study programmes will integrate time spent in ward rounds, case conferences, academic courses, 'self-help' groups and self-study. Notes on the most commonly used reference books for MRCPsych are included.

The exam papers seek to give a guide to the level of difficulty of the actual examinations. The questions were designed to be as representative as possible. We hope that the exam papers can be used as tolerable practice exams under examination conditions and times. Practice in Multiple-Choice Question (MCQ) technique is vital in examinations where negative marking is to be used. Candidates often fear losing marks by answering too many questions, when a simple truth is that unless they answer more than 90% or so of the questions they will simply fail to gain adequate marks. A breadth of reading is required for all the MCQ examinations. No single text is sufficient. Candidates in the Part II examinations are often surprised by the content of the MCQ examinations, particularly concerning the Basic Sciences paper.

The choice of questions in the actual examination has been criticised for irrelevance by both trainees and trainers. Despite this, the general approach of the College is fair enough and some thought can usually prove the relevance of all the questions. That they often seem obscure or difficult is a reflection of the fact that the production of questions able to differentiate between highly selected and trained candidates is no easy task.

The MCQs are followed by answer sections that include true/false answers, often accompanied by extended explanations, with references. We have chosen the references carefully to cover many classic papers. Tracking them down and reading them will pay dividends.

Specifically for the Part II we have included an example Short Answer Question (SAQ) paper, six Patient Management Problems (PMPs), and a sample Essay paper.

The Clinical Examination is the hurdle that brings down most candidates since a pass in this section is mandatory for both parts of the MRCPsych. There is no rigid, 'right' way to approach this part of the exam. However, there are classic pitfalls to avoid. Our section on clinical exams will help you to avoid them! A key element of success is to appear safe and conventional. No marks are awarded for radical heroism. An awareness of organic factors and a salient physical examination are held in high esteem, but will need to be counter-balanced by an adequate awareness of the psychological factors operating in your particular patient.

Finally, we have striven to exclude any errors, but as you will appreciate there is much detail in the book. We would be grateful for any constructive comments or suggestions that interested readers may make to help us improve future editions.

Ben Green, 1993

List of contributors

Dr David Anderson FRCPsych
Consultant Psychiatrist and Associate Medical Director
Mersey Care NHS Trust

Dr Simon Bainbridge MRCPsych
Staff Grade Psychiatrist
Cheadle Royal Hospital

Dr Kay Callender MRCPsych
Consultant Psychiatrist in Eating Disorders
Cheadle Royal Hospital

Dr Eric Davies BSc (Hons), MB, ChB (Hons), PhD, MRCPsych
Specialist Registrar in Child and Adolescent Psychiatry
Honorary Research Fellow
University of Manchester

Dr Lesley Faith MRCPsych
Consultant in Psychiatric Intensive Care
Cheadle Royal Hospital

Dr Tim Morris MB, ChB, MRCPsych, MSc
Consultant Child Psychiatrist
Honorary Lecturer in Psychiatry
Burnley General Hospital

Dr Deep Majumdar MRCPsych
Consultant Psychiatrist
Mersey Care NHS Trust

Professor Chris McWilliams
Consultant Psychiatrist
Ribbleton Hospital, Preston

Dr Natasha Walford MRCPsych
Specialist Registrar in Psychiatry
Queen's Park Hospital, Blackburn

Professor Ken Wilson
Division of Psychiatry
University of Liverpool

Some material has been derived from the first and second editions of this book and the contributors are noted in previous editions.

To Dominic, my son.

The MRCPsych Study Programme

Ben Green

It is important for you to design your own programme to boost your chances of success at Membership because everybody studies in their own way. You will need to give consideration to acquiring both the knowledge and skills necessary to pass the MRCPsych and, since the exam also seeks to establish whether you are acquiring the necessary skills to be a consultant, working towards the exam will complement your general training.

These skills are developed in your clinical attachment as General Professional Trainees and for reference's sake some of these are listed in Box 1.

Box 1 Clinical competencies of senior house officers (SHOs)

The following list of skills and competencies are those that many consultants would expect an SHO to learn and foster.

- Ability to assess a patient and produce a safe and relevant management plan.
- Ability to assess risk of suicide.
- Ability to assess risk of dangerousness to others.
- Familiarity with, and appropriate use of, the Mental Health Act.
- Management of a case of severe depressive disorder.
- Management of a case of first-episode psychosis.
- Management of a case of schizophrenia.
- Management of a case of anxiety.
- Management of a case of alcohol withdrawal, delirium and/or dependence.
- Management of a case of substance abuse, delirium and/or dependence.
- Management of a case of bipolar affective disorder.
- Safe management of the disturbed patient.

- Assessment and management of a case of dementia.
- Familiarity with, and appropriate use of, a modern classification system.
- Management of a case of anxiety disorder.
- Management of a case of obsessive compulsive disorder.
- Management of a case of post-traumatic stress disorder.
- Assess a patient appropriately for and referral of a patient to a specialist psychotherapy service.
- Assess a patient appropriately for and referral of a patient to a specialist forensic service.
- Assess a patient appropriately for and referral of a patient to a specialist child and adolescent service.
- Assess a patient appropriately for and referral of a patient to a specialist learning disability service.
- See a short-term patient for a supervised form of psychotherapy.
- See a long-term patient for a supervised form of psychotherapy.
- Safely and effectively administer a course of ECT (electroconvulsive therapy).
- Familiarity with collateral legislation with relevance to psychiatric practice such as the Children's Act.
- Familiarity with, and appropriate use of, the leadership role in the multidisciplinary team.
- Familiarity with relevant modern-day business and management techniques.
- Familiarity with management guidelines and systems such as the Care Programme Approach (CPA).
- Safely practise breakaway techniques and approved self-defence skills.
- Devise protocols for clinical audit and also for academic research.
- Ability to liaise appropriately with statutory bodies such as the Mental Health Act Commission.
- Ability to appear and speak at Mental Health Act tribunals, where appropriate.
- Ability to interview patients for, and write, satisfactory legal and official reports.
- Satisfactorily perform cardiopulmonary resuscitation.
- Familiarity with information technology (IT) systems to the benefit of patient care and research skills.
- Ability to liaise effectively, courteously and appropriately with professional colleagues involved in the multidisciplinary care of patients.

- Ability to introspect about and gain insight from the doctor–patient relationship.
- Ability to communicate effectively with patients, colleagues and groups.
- Ability to teach effectively.

Although some people appear to relish leaving everything until the last moment, such 'binge working' can lead to panic in the exam. In any event the gains in terms of study are rapidly lost after 'binge working' since the knowledge base is poorly rehearsed. The best method is to develop a programme where you can daily eat away at gaining the knowledge and skills required. The College has certain conditions it sets before trainees can sit its exams. The College stipulates minimum times that must be spent on approved psychiatric training schemes. Before candidates can sit MRCPsych Part I they must have spent one year training on such a scheme.

In 2005 the College website stated:

'Applicants must have completed twelve months of post-registration full-time training (or equivalent part-time, flexible training) in posts approved by the Royal College of Psychiatrists, by the date of the Written Paper Examination. This must be made up as follows:
- twelve months of General Adult Psychiatry; *or*
- six months of General Adult Psychiatry *and* six months of Old Age Psychiatry.'

The MRCPsych Part II candidate must have passed Part I and spent at least two years full-time in approved post-registration training.

In 2005 the College website stated about MRCPsych Part II:

'Candidates must have passed, or have been granted exemption from, the MRCPsych Part I Examination, and have completed *thirty* months of full-time post-registration training (or equivalent part-time flexible training) in posts approved by the Royal College of Psychiatrists, by the date of the written papers. This must be made up as follows, and includes training undertaken towards MRCPsych Part I:
- twelve months (minimum) in General Adult Psychiatry; *and*
- eighteen months in any psychiatric sub-speciality (including General Adult) but no more than twelve months in any one such sub-speciality (apart from General Adult).
The duration of any one training post must not be less than six months, and training must be supported by a concurrent academic course.'

With regard to re-sitting the Part II exam the 2005 College website says:

> 'All trainees who fail the MRCPsych Part II Examination at the *first attempt* may apply for a second attempt without undergoing further training, but they must still fulfil the requirements in terms of Registration and Sponsorship.
>
>   *Full-time trainees and Flexible (part-time) trainees entering for their third or subsequent attempts:* Candidates are required to re-enter or remain in approved psychiatric training, which is supported by an appropriate academic course or programme of education and clinical instruction approved by the applicant's College Tutor, between the second and third and each subsequent attempt at the Examination. This further training may be in any psychiatric sub-speciality.'

In addition the candidate's consultant and clinical tutor must confirm attendance at an academic course on his or her sponsorship forms. The College states that attendance at such a course must be 75% of the time. However, even 100% attendance at one of these academic courses does not automatically confer the ability to take the exam and pass. The course, like this study manual, will only work for you if you can put in additional time and energy: gathering knowledge through reading books and papers, attending case conferences/journal clubs, and seeing patients and formally presenting them (to exam standard).

   The candidate must also be able to support their application to sit the exam with two sponsors, so that each application for the examination must be supported by statements from two consultant psychiatrists who are subscribing Members or Fellows of the Royal College of Psychiatrists. The first sponsor must be the applicant's College tutor, and the second sponsor must be a consultant psychiatrist who has supervised the applicant's training for at least four months in the year prior to the closing date for receipt of applications. It is courteous and wise to approach consultants *before* citing them as sponsors.

   The format of the exams is as follows:

MRCPsych Part I
The Part I Examination has two components:

1   One Written Paper – Individual Statements and Extended Matching Items (90 minutes – 133 Individual Statements and 30 Extended Matching Items).
2   One Clinical Examination – the Objective Structured Clinical Examination (OSCE).

MRCPsych Part II
The Part II Examination has four components:

1   TWO Written Papers (each 165 Individual Statements and 15 Extended Matching Items – 90 minutes):
    ● Sciences basic to psychiatry
    ● Clinical Topics.
2   Essay Paper (90 minutes).
3   Critical Review Paper (90 minutes).
4   Clinical Examinations:
    ● Individual Patient Assessment
    ● Patient Management Problems (30 minutes).

The temptation to take the exam as soon as possible is understandable, but caution should be exercised. Extra experience is always valuable in the clinical components. Although an early pass (through taking the exam as soon as possible) can be advantageous in career terms, an early fail can be a blot on the CV (especially at the Part I level). Waiting until you are well prepared will enhance morale when you eventually take the exam.

At Part I only those candidates who pass the Written Paper will be permitted to take the Clinical Examination.

As of 2005 the limit on the number of attempts that candidates can make at the MRCPsych Part I has been removed by decision of the Court of Electors. Any candidate who can satisfy the eligibility requirements for entry to the examination, as specified in the Regulations, will therefore be allowed to do so. This includes those candidates previously deemed as Final Fail candidates. No further Final Fail notifications will now be issued.

Given the above arguments you can see the desirability of starting your study programme as early as you can. Candidates for Part I who read this book will presumably go on to be candidates for Part II, and so all the advice below is relevant in attaining your long-term goal. A small amount of time set aside each day for this long-term goal will pay real dividends in your final revision.

Key strategies for the MRCPsych Study Programme

1   You will need at least one large text for the exam. Since none of the available texts is comprehensive you may need to find two. Unfortunately they are expensive, but they usually give a consistent and balanced overview which, hopefully, will accord with the views of your examiners. Check with

booksellers that you are buying the latest edition, or that a new edition is not about to appear in the next few weeks.

2 Think in terms of the exam while you work. For instance, if you're coming up for Part II, when you're in a ward round or in clinic, analyse how your consultants manage their patients. All too often trainees adopt a 'cross-sectional' view of a patient. The immediate mental state is important, but a longitudinal view takes experience to evolve. Match your own ideas for management against those of senior trainees and consultants. Such a policy will make the Patient Management Problems (PMPs) easier.

3 View the group training activities in your hospital, such as journal clubs and case conferences, as valuable training opportunities rather than imposed chores. Use what helpful feedback is given to you on your presentation, but don't be disheartened by any negative feedback. By rights all criticisms should be constructive, but sometimes in such case-conference audiences there is an individual who enjoys looking superior. Test what they have to say, but don't let them destroy your confidence!

4 Start building up a library of useful classic papers that you have read or heard presented. You will need to organise these in some way so that you can use them efficiently in your revision. Depending upon how obsessional you are you could distil the ideas that are most relevant and put them on a card index (or in a computer database). The exam will probably not focus on individual papers, but on a body of knowledge. However, well-replicated studies may feature. Putting detailed references in your essay could be impressive if they are right and well chosen, but they may be just irritating if they are wrong or spurious and will not enhance your paper. Read a few journals regularly. Review articles in the *British Journal of Psychiatry* and *Psychological Medicine* can be useful guides for further study.

5 Both at Part I and Part II levels gather an informal group of colleagues who are all studying for the exam, and organise yourselves to hear each other's case presentations and quiz each other on diagnosis (according to ICD-10 categories) and management issues. Not only will this give invaluable practice for the exam, but will also produce a ready-made self-help group. The group needs to form at least several months before the exam. So that the group doesn't get into bad habits (e.g. all the group might be labouring under some misapprehension about exam technique), inject some outside ideas by inviting along a specialist registrar with the Membership or a consultant to check presentation skills. Several university MRCPsych courses (e.g. Liverpool) are now using small groups and problem-based learning techniques to enhance presentation skills and develop self-learning strategies.

6 If there is a local consultant who is also a College examiner at Part I or Part II level do try to draw on their expertise. Ask them to coach you and to hear you present cases you have seen under exam conditions.

7 Either as an individual or as a group try to gain access to a video camera to record you as you present. Your local College tutor should be able to arrange access to a video camera for this purpose. There may be things that you do completely unconsciously that seriously detract from the observer's confidence in you as a clinician. A slumped posture may convey an uncaring approach to the patient. Putting your hand in front of your mouth may affect what the examiners hear of your presentation. Lack of eye contact with the examiners may make you appear unduly schizoid! Video feedback can help you change your presentation for the better and as you see the positive effects of that change on subsequent tapes your confidence will be boosted enormously. Tapes of you interviewing the patient can draw out valuable information on your interviewing style and content.

8 Set aside a regular time each day for study and reviewing how your study programme is going. It is easy to ignore long-term goals while you are taking care of short-term demands on your time and energy. Before you know it, the opportunities for fulfilling your long-term goals have gone and only panic measures are left. The time you spend each day needn't be excessive (you should aim to enjoy the time you spend studying, thereby reinforcing the behaviour), but it should be 'protected', i.e. without interruptions, and at a regular time, and when you are not too tired.

9 Although having attended an academic course is seen as an essential requirement for sitting Part I and Part II, it is a fact that courses in different regions vary and that your individual attitude to the course will also vary. Some courses set out with the explicit aim of getting you through Membership, while others gear themselves towards generating skills and research. All these approaches are valid in that they will further your training, but you will need to adapt to the kind of course your region runs, profit by its strengths and rectify its weaknesses through your own endeavour. Try to interact with the course as far as you can. Look through the programme for the weeks ahead and consider adapting your individual study to complement it. Perhaps you could read the literature on operant and classical conditioning around the time that there is course teaching on the psychology of learning. Ask and answer questions during the course teaching. Don't be afraid to make a mistake; you are checking whether you've understood the subject thoroughly.

10 Well in advance of the exam write to the Royal College to obtain the most up-to-date details of the exam and available past papers. Over time the exam does change, and hopefully evolve. There is now a 'syllabus' of sorts, which is available from the College. Make sure you have the most up-to-date copy you can find.

11 Ask colleagues which books they are currently using and what they think of them. Below are several suggestions with some comments of recommendation.

Texts

There are numerous pocket handbooks that offer advice in clinical situations. Some pocket handbooks that seem better than the rest are:

● Goldberg D and Murray R (2002) *The Maudsley Handbook of Practical Psychiatry*. Oxford Medical Publications, Oxford.
● Jacobson JL and Jacobson AM (2000) *Psychiatric Secrets*. Hanley & Belfus Inc, Philadelphia.
● Puri BK and McKee H (1998) *A Psychiatric Vade-Mecum*. Arnold, London.

See also:

● Lader M, Kerwin R and Checkley S (2005) *Handbook of Psychopharmacology: The Maudsley Handbook*. Sage Publications, London.

Standard-style texts include:

● Gelder M, Lopez-Ibor J and Andreasen N (2003) *New Oxford Textbook of Psychiatry*. Oxford University Press, Oxford. (Eminently readable, balanced text, recently expanded. Most suited to Part I.)
● Lawrie S, Owens D, Sharpe M *et al.* (2004) *Companion to Psychiatric Studies*. Churchill Livingstone, Edinburgh. (Good all-round and in-depth cover of topics. Most applicable to Part II.)
● Puri BK and Tyrer PJ (1998) *Sciences Basic to Psychiatry* (2e). Churchill Livingstone, Edinburgh. (Useful for Part I and Basic Sciences MCQ paper of MRCPsych Part II. Second edition now probably slightly dated.)

Organic psychiatry

The general texts above will need to be supplemented by a specialised text such as:

● Lishman WA (1998) *Organic Psychiatry* (3e). Blackwell Scientific Publications, Oxford.
● Yudofsky SC and Hales RE (2002) *The American Psychiatric Press Textbook of Neuropsychiatry*. American Psychiatric Press, Arlington, VA. (Highly recommended.)

Diagnostic classification

The tenth version of the International Classification of Diseases is mandatory reading for both parts of the exam. You will need to acquire your own copy for frequent reference.

● World Health Organization (WHO) (1994) *Pocket Guide to the ICD-10 Classification*. Churchill Livingstone, Edinburgh. (The guide is based on: World Health Organization (1992) *The ICD-10 Classification of Mental and Behavioural Disorders. Clinical descriptions and diagnostic guidelines. 10th edition*. World Health Organization, Geneva.)

For completeness I also mention the American Psychiatric Association's DSM-IV system which has become progressively similar to the WHO system over the years. The *DSM-IV Casebook* is useful for the clinical examinations; it contains a vast range of case vignettes that are followed by expert discussions and differential diagnoses.

● American Psychiatric Association (2000) *Diagnostic and Statistical Manual of Mental Disorders: DSM-IV-TR: fourth edition text revision*. American Psychiatric Publishing Inc, Arlington, VA.
● Spitzer RL *et al*. (2002) *DSM-IV-TR Casebook: a learning companion to the Diagnostic and Statistical Manual of Mental Disorders*. American Psychiatric Publishing Inc, Arlington, VA. (Interesting to read the cases and see whether you can figure out the correct diagnosis – therefore useful for Part I and Part II clinical exams and also PMPs. However, be well aware of any differences with respect to ICD-10.)

Psychopathology

For the Part I clinical exam a thorough knowledge of psychopathology is essential. General textbooks like those above inevitably have a section on symptoms and signs, but for the purposes of the exam an investment in a specific text is worthwhile.

The contemporary book is Professor Sims' *Symptoms in the Mind*.

● Sims A (2002) *Symptoms in the Mind: an introduction to descriptive psychopathology*. Baillière Tindall, London.

The classic text for some time used to be Liverpool's Professor Fish's *Clinical Psychopathology*, which although at times wordy and abstruse had some real insights. Karl Jaspers' *General Psychopathology* was published by Manchester University Press in 1963, but has sadly gone out of print, so that copies can only be viewed in libraries. This large book is fascinating to read for its breadth and its philosophy as much as anything. References to Jaspers' work have occurred in both parts of the MRCPsych examination.

For those fascinated by psychopathology and the underlying neurology and psychology we also suggest a book edited by EMR Critchley, *The Neurological Boundaries of Reality* (1994), published by Jason Aronson.

In both clinical exams you will be observed interviewing a patient. The questions you ask patients obviously condition their responses. The examiners will be interested in how well you interact with your patient. It is advisable to use standardised forms of questions such as those in the Present State Examination (Wing *et al.*, 1974, 1987) or the Geriatric Mental State Examination (Copeland *et al.*, 1976, 1988). *Psychiatric Examination in Clinical Practice* by Leff and Isaacs covers basic aspects of the psychiatric assessment, but is weak on cognitive examination.

A book that now covers both interviewing techniques and also psychopathology is *Psychiatric Interviewing* (2nd edition) by Shea. There is a bias in the book towards the US Board examinations, but nevertheless the generic advice is extremely sound and it can be thoroughly recommended.

An alternative shorter book on the psychiatric interview is *A Guide to Psychiatric Examination* by Aquilina and Warner (2004), which is perhaps stronger on the features of organic presentations and the adaptations necessary in the cognitive section of the Mental State Examination.

- Aquilina C and Warner J (2004) *A Guide to Psychiatric Examination*. Pastest, Knutsford.
- Copeland JRM *et al.* (1976) A semi-structured clinical interview for the assessment of diagnosis and mental state in the elderly: the Geriatric Mental State Schedule. 1. Development and reliability. *Psychological Medicine*. 6: 439–49.
- Copeland JRM *et al.* (1988) The Geriatric Mental State and AGECAT diagnosis in community studies. *Psychological Medicine*. 8: 219–23.
- Critchley EMR (1994) *The Neurological Boundaries of Reality*. Jason Aronson, New York.
- Fish F (1967) *Clinical Psychopathology*. Wright, Bristol.
- Jaspers K (1963) *General Psychopathology*. Manchester University Press, Manchester.
- Shea SC (1998) *Psychiatric Interviewing. The art of understanding*. Saunders, Philadelphia.
- Wing JK, Cooper JE and Sartorius N (1974) *The Description of Psychiatric Symptoms: an introduction manual for the PSE and CATEGO system*. Cambridge University Press, Cambridge.
- Wing JK *et al.* (1987) Further developments of the 'Present State Examination' and CATEGO system. *Archives of Psychiatry and Neurological Sciences*. **22**: 151–60.

Psychotherapy

Individual Statement questions, PMPs and Essays often focus on the scientific basis for psychotherapy, and it is therefore wise to have a thorough knowledge of recent research.

- Bergin A, Garfield S and Lambert M (2003) *Bergin and Garfield's Handbook of Psychotherapy and Behavior Change*. John Wiley and Sons, New York. (Interesting and comprehensive account of psychotherapy research.)
- Gopfert M *et al*. (2004) *Parental Psychiatric Disorder: distressed parents and their families*. Cambridge University Press, Cambridge. (Excellent account of this vital area.)
- Hawton K *et al*. (1999) *Cognitive Behaviour Therapy for Psychiatric Problems: a practical guide*. Oxford University Press, Oxford. (Well-written and concise. Tells you all you need to know to be able to start cognitive therapy. Since cognitive therapy can often appear rather mysterious it is pleasing to read such a helpful book. Useful if you are asked in OSCEs, PMP, or Essays to explain stages in cognitive therapy.)
- Malan DH (1995) *Individual Psychotherapy and the Science of Psychodynamics*. Butterworth-Heinemann, London. (Comprehensible account of psychodynamic psychotherapy with clear case examples.)
- Ryle A and Kerr I (2002) *Introducing Cognitive Analytic Therapy: principles and practice*. John Wiley and Sons, London.
- Yalom I and Leszcz M (2005) *Theory and Practice of Group Psychotherapy*. Basic Books, New York.

Neuroanatomy, neurophysiology and neurology

A good working knowledge of neurology, neurophysiology and the neuroanatomy behind clinical examination is essential for both parts of the exam.

- Carpenter RHS (2002) *Neurophysiology*. Hodder Arnold, London. Book and disk. (All you ever wished to know about neurophysiology and an atlas of neuroanatomy as well.)
- Ginsberg L (2004) *Lecture Notes On Neurology*. Blackwell Publishing, Oxford.
- Malhi G, Matharu M and Hale A (2000) *Neurology for Psychiatrists*. Dunitz, London.
- Martin JH (2003) *Neuroanatomy*. Appleton and Lange Publishers, Stamford. (Describes neuroanatomy quite lucidly and includes analysis of function and behaviours as well. Includes MRI – magnetic resonance imaging – and other scans.)

Research methods

Details of research methods feature in the Part II Basic Sciences MCQs. More extended descriptions of research and statistical methods regularly feature as Essays and in the Critical Review Paper.

- Brown T and Wilkinson G (2005) *Critical Reviews in Psychiatry*. Royal College of Psychiatrists Seminar Series. Gaskell, London.
- Freeman C (1995) *Research Methods in Psychiatry: a beginner's guide* (2e). American Psychiatric Press, Arlington, VA. (The best text available in this field at Membership level. Comprehensive and interesting.)
- Lawrie S, McIntosh A and Rao S (2000) *Critical Appraisal for Psychiatrists*. Churchill Livingstone, Edinburgh.
- Roberts M and Ilardi S (2005) *Handbook of Research Methods in Clinical Psychology*. Blackwell Publishing, Oxford. (Looks at experimental and quasi-experimental designs, statistical analysis, validity, ethics, cultural diversity, and the scientific process of publishing.)

In terms of biostatistics there is now a wealth of very useful books from the simple handbook type to more detailed works. Suggestions include:

- Norman GR and Streiner GL (2003) *PDQ Stratistics*. BC Decker Publishers, Burlington.

Mental Health Act

- Department of Health and Welsh Office (1999) *Code of Practice. Mental Health Act 1983*. HMSO, London. (English and Welsh candidates may find the Code a useful resource. If you introduce concepts from the Code in discussions in Patient Management Problems and Clinical it will give the impression that you have a good and up-to-date working knowledge of the Act.)
- Jones R (2004) *Mental Health Act Manual*. Sweet and Maxwell, London. (Not totally user-friendly, but a definitive guide that is often to be seen on the table at mental health tribunals – probably mainly for the pedants.)

Substance abuse

- Alcoholics Anonymous (2002) *Big Book* (4e). Hazelden Publishing and Educational Services, Center City.
- Chick J and Cantwell R (1994) *Seminars in Alcohol and Drug Misuse*. College seminars. Gaskell (Royal College of Psychiatrists), London.

- Edwards G *et al.* (1994) *Alcohol Policy and the Public Good.* Oxford University Press, Oxford.
- Ghodse H (2002) *Drugs and Addictive Behaviour: a guide to treatment.* Blackwell, Oxford.
- Heather N and Robertson I (1997) *Problem Drinking.* Oxford University Press, Oxford.

Learning disability

- Fraser W and Kerr M (2003) *Seminars in the Psychiatry of Learning Disability.* College seminars. Gaskell (Royal College of Psychiatrists), London.

Journals and papers

Read the following journals regularly:

- *Acta Psychiatrica Scandinavica*
- *American Journal of Psychiatry*
- *Archives of General Psychiatry*
- *British Journal of Psychiatry*
- *Current Opinion in Psychiatry*
- *Psychological Medicine.*

Obtain copies of the rather daunting College reading lists (published for various subject headings) and read at least some of the references.

The review articles in *Psychological Medicine* are worth spending a lot of time on. The Part II Essay paper often reflects the general scope of these reviews.

Read the quality national press as well for articles on healthcare provision. Essays before now have used quotes from health ministers and editorials. The purpose of such informal study would not be to 'spot' questions, but to give you some general ammunition for such articles on debates in psychiatric care provision.

History of psychiatry

Some questions feature historical perspectives or information and some knowledge of the history of psychiatry can be interesting as well as essential for the exam.

- Healy D (1996, 1998) *The Psychopharmacologists*. Volumes 1 and 2. Arnold, London.
- Porter R (1990) *Mind-Forg'd Manacles*. Penguin, London.

Psychology

A psychology text appears to be essential for the Membership exam at both Parts I and II.

- Gleitman H (2003) *Psychology*. WW Norton and Company, New York.
- Smith E *et al.* (2002) *Atkinson and Hilgard's Introduction to Psychology*. Wadsworth, Belmont. (Easily read texts for psychology undergraduates. Check for latest edition since fairly regularly updated.)
- McCarthy RA and Warrington EK (1990) *Cognitive Neuropsychology: a clinical introduction*. Academic Press, London.
- Schultz D and Schultz SE (2004) *Theories of Personality*. Wadsworth, Belmont. (An excellent guide to various personality theories – highly recommended.)

Try also guides such as Penguin's *Dictionary of Psychology*, which contains a smattering of information on diverse topics enabling you to associate concepts with famous names and schools of psychology – a useful strategy for MCQ-type questions.

Psychopharmacology

- Cookson J, Taylor D and Katona C (2002) *Use of Drugs in Psychiatry: the evidence from psychopharmacology*. Gaskell, London.
- Green B (2004) *Focus on Antipsychotics*. Petroc Press, Newbury.
- Haddad P, Dursun S and Deakin B (2004) *Adverse Syndromes and Psychiatric Drugs: a clinical guide*. Oxford University Press, Oxford.
- Healy D (2001) *Psychiatric Drugs Explained*. Churchill Livingstone, Edinburgh.
- Stahl SM and Grady MM (2004) *Essential Psychopharmacology: the prescriber's guide*. Cambridge University Press, Cambridge.

Liaison psychiatry

- Guthrie E and Creed F (1996) *Seminars in Liaison Psychiatry*. Royal College of Psychiatrists, Gaskell, London. (Essential Part II reading.

Reasonable coverage of the area and up to date, concise – useful for references.)

- Royal College of Psychiatrists (1994) *The General Hospital Management of Adult Deliberate Self Harm*. Report CR32. Royal College of Psychiatrists, London. (A consensus statement on standards of service provision in relation to deliberate self-harm.)
- Royal College of Psychiatrists and Royal College of Physicians (1992) *Medical Symptoms Not Explained by Organic Disease*. Royal College of Psychiatrists and Royal College of Physicians, London. (Examines the area of 'unexplained' medical symptoms such as irritable bowel disorder, chronic fatigue syndrome, atypical chest pain and describes management strategies in the light of current research findings.)
- Royal College of Psychiatrists and Royal College of Physicians (1995) *The Psychological Care of Medical Patients – recognition of need and service provision*. Report CR 35. Royal College of Psychiatrists and Royal College of Physicians, London. (Essential reading for Part II. Short, easily read, describes different models, prevalence, classification of disorders encountered in medical settings, and problems and suggestions for service provision. Also useful source of references.)
- Royal College of Psychiatrists and Royal College of Physicians (1995) *Psychiatric Aspects of Physical Disease*. Royal College of Psychiatrists and Royal College of Physicians, London. (Accompanies the above report, goes into further details of relationship, prevalence. Also gives examples of services, disorders and management in the area of HIV [human immunodeficiency virus] and AIDS [acquired immune deficiency syndrome], stroke, cancer care, coronary artery disease and diabetes. Again, is short and easily read.)
- Society for Psychosomatic Research (1993) *Psychological Treatment in Disease and Illness*. Gaskell, London. (Discusses development in psychological treatments for 'psychosomatic' disorders in the light of current research findings.)

Sociology and social psychiatry

An elementary knowledge of sociology with regard to medicine is essential for Part II. Concepts such as stigma, institutionalisation, social class, race, culture, and sociological views on the family and society are bread-and-butter stuff and key reference papers should be thoroughly explored and essential details memorised.

- Bhugra D and Leff J (1993) *Principles of Social Psychiatry*. Blackwell, Oxford.

- Brown G and Harris TO (1978) *Social Origins of Depression*. Tavistock, London.
- Goffman E (1961) *Asylums: essays on the social situation of mental patients and other inmates*. Penguin, Harmondsworth. (*See also* his work on stigma.)
- Goldberg D and Huxley P (1980) *Mental Illness in the Community*. Tavistock, London.
- Pilgrim D and Rogers A (1993) *A Sociology of Mental Health and Illness*. Open University Press, Buckingham.
- Prior L (1993) *The Social Organisation of Mental Illness*. Sage, London.
- Scambler G (1991) *Sociology As Applied To Medicine* (3e). Baillière Tindall, London.

Child and adolescent psychiatry

Goodman and Scott's *Child Psychiatry* is a useful introductory text, but lacks sufficient depth, particularly in terms of research detail. The alternative is the comprehensive but now slightly elderly tome by Rutter, Hersov and Taylor.

- Goodman R and Scott S (2005) *Child Psychiatry*. Blackwell, Oxford.
- Lask B, Taylor S and Nunn K (2003) *Practical Child Psychiatry. The clinician's guide*. BMJ Books, London.
- Rutter M, Hersov L and Taylor E (1995) *Child and Adolescent Psychiatry: modern approaches*. Blackwell Science, Oxford.

Forensic psychiatry

As with child psychiatry it is difficult to find texts that are precisely suitable. Most fall into the traps of being either too simple or too long/complicated and thus too expensive. Bearing in mind these constraints I can suggest the following:

- Bluglass R and Bowden P (eds) (1990) *Principles and Practice of Forensic Psychiatry*. Churchill Livingstone, London.
- Chiswick D and Cope R (1995) *Seminars in Forensic Psychiatry*. Royal College of Psychiatrists, Gaskell, London.
- Gunn J and Taylor PJ (1993) *Forensic Psychiatry. Clinical, legal and ethical issues*. Butterworth Heinemann, Oxford.
- O'Shea K *et al.* (1999) *Faulk's Basic Forensic Psychiatry*. Blackwell, Oxford.

MRCPsych Part I: MCQ Written Paper

Individual Statements

---

1 Rett syndrome occurs in both boys and girls.

2 According to ICD-10 violence confined to family members is not one of the signs of conduct disorder.

3 Transitional objects are associated with the work of Bowlby.

4 Being female is associated with slower speech development.

5 Conduct disorder is present in less than 3% of boys aged under 10.

---

1 True.

Although it predominantly affects girls, occurring in 1 in every 10 000 to 15 000 female births, it does occur rarely in boys. The fault has recently been pinpointed to the MeCP2 gene on the X chromosome. Recurrence in the same family is very rare – Rett syndrome is sporadic in most cases.

Reference:

- Amir RE *et al*. (2000) Influence of mutation type and X chromosome inactivation on Rett syndrome phenotypes. *Annals of Neurology*. 47(5): 670–9.

2 False.

One of the conduct disorders described in ICD-10 is *F91.0 Conduct Disorder Confined to the Family Context* in which violence against family members (but not others) and deliberate fire setting, among other signs, are grounds for the diagnosis.

3 False.

Transitional objects are associated with the work of Winnicott.

4 False.

Being female is associated with earlier and better speech development.

5 False.

Conduct disorder was found in 4% of boys studied by Rutter *et al.* in the classic Isle of Wight Study. Other studies have found rates even higher to about 16%.

Reference:

- Rutter M, Tizard J, Yule W, Graham P and Whitmore K (1976) Research report: Isle of Wight Studies, 1964–1974. *Psychological Medicine.* **6**(2): 313–32.

6 Increasing rates of childhood psychiatric disorders can in part be explained by changes in social acceptability.

7 Quetiapine causes gynaecomastia.

8 SSRIs prescribed in pregnancy are associated with reduced birth weight.

9 Drugs that can cause depression include tetrabanazine.

10 Drugs that can induce psychosis include mefloquine.

6 True.

7 False.

Gynaecomastia is associated with hyperprolactinaemia secondary to some antipsychotics as prolactin is under the inhibitory control of dopamine. Quetiapine however does not usually raise prolactin levels. Neither does clozapine or aripiprazole.

Reference:

- Taylor D, Paton C and Kerwin R (2005) *Maudsley 2005–2006 Prescribing Guidelines.* Taylor and Francis, London.

8 True.

SSRIs (selective serotonin reuptake inhibitors) prescribed in pregnancy are associated with reduced birth weight and also reduced gestational age (although depression itself is associated with reduced gestational age). SSRIs are not generally believed to be teratogenic.

Reference:

- Taylor D, Paton C and Kerwin R (2005) *Maudsley 2005–2006 Prescribing Guidelines.* Taylor and Francis, London.

9 True.

10 True.
Mefloquine can indeed cause psychosis, but this seems uncommon. The incidence rate of psychosis during current mefloquine exposure has been calculated as 1.0/1000 person-years.

References:

- Meier CR, Wilcock K and Jick SS (2004) The risk of severe depression, psychosis or panic attacks with prophylactic antimalarials. *Drug Safety.* **27**(3): 203–13.
- Stuiver PC, Ligthelm RJ and Goud TJ (1989) Acute psychosis after mefloquine. [Letter.] *The Lancet.* **2**(8657): 282.

---

11 Post-traumatic stress disorder (PTSD) must arise within four months of the traumatic event for an ICD-10 diagnosis.

12 De Clerambault's syndrome usually involves a delusion of infidelity.

13 *Echo de la pensees* is the experience of hearing one's thoughts simultaneously spoken out loud.

14 Charles Bonnet syndrome involves complex visual hallucinations.

15 Parapraxis is a difficulty with dressing associated with parietal lobe damage.

---

11 **False.**
ICD-10 guidelines acknowledge that there may be a latency period between the trauma and the onset of PTSD, but say that this rarely exceeds six months. Nevertheless the diagnosis may still be possible if the onset is after six months if the clinical manifestations are feasible.

Reference:

- World Health Organization (1992) *ICD-10 Clinical Descriptions and Diagnostic Guidelines.* WHO, Geneva.

12 **False.**
De Clerambault (1872–1934) was a French psychiatrist. He is known for the syndrome in which patients believe themselves to be the object of attention or love of a famous or unattainable person such as a king or film star. The delusion of infidelity or morbid jealousy is associated with the Othello syndrome.

13 False.

Gedankenlautwerden is the experience of hearing one's thoughts simultaneously spoken out loud. *Echo de la pensees* is the experience of hearing one's thoughts spoken out loud after a slight delay, not simultaneously.

14 True.

Charles Bonnet syndrome involves complex visual hallucinations. It is sometimes seen in the elderly and in patients with central or peripheral impairment/loss of vision.

15 False.

Parapraxis is a term coined for a Freudian slip of the tongue. Dressing dyspraxia is a difficulty with dressing associated with parietal lobe damage.

---

16 'Knifeblade' atrophy on brain scan is a recognised feature of Wilson's disease (hepatolenticular degeneration).

17 Bereavement increases the risks of subsequent depressive disorder and also death.

18 Tardive dyskinesia can be measured using the Abnormal Involuntary Movements Scale.

19 Pareidolia is classified as a symptom of psychosis.

20 Psychological defence mechanisms are usually associated with the work of Reich.

---

16 False.

Wilson's disease results from an abnormally low serum caeruloplasmin level, and consequently high serum copper levels so that there is a resulting deposition of copper in the CNS (central nervous system) and elsewhere. Diagnosis is by measuring caeruloplasmin levels and testing urine collections for the excess urinary excretion of copper. Wilson's disease has an autosomal recessive inheritance. 'Knifeblade' atrophy is characteristically seen in Pick's disease.

Reference:

- Lishman WA (1998) *Organic Psychiatry* (3e). Blackwell, London.

17 True.

Klerman and Izen (1977) reviewed various studies and concluded that there was an increased mortality which peaked in the second six months after bereavement.

References:

- Green BH, Copeland JR, Dewey ME, Sharma V, Saunders PA, Davidson IA, Sullivan C and McWilliam C (1992) Risk factors for depression in elderly people: a prospective study. *Acta Psychiatrica Scandinavica*. 86(3): 213–17.
- Klerman GL and Izen JE (1977) The effect of bereavement and grief on physical health and general well-being. *Adv Psychosomat Med*. 9: 63–104.

18 True.

Reference:

- Smith JM, Kucharski LT, Eblen C, Knutsen E and Linn C (1979) An assessment of tardive dyskinesia in schizophrenic outpatients. *Psychopharmacology*. 64(1): 99–104.

19 False.
Pareidolia is where ill-defined sense impressions (e.g. staring into the fire) conjure up ill-formed and fleeting images.

Reference:

- Fish F (1967) *Clinical Psychopathology*. Wright, Bristol.

20 False.
Defence mechanisms were elaborated by Sigmund Freud and his daughter, Anna. The work of Melanie Klein is also associated with defence mechanisms.

---

21 Paradoxical injunction is associated with the work of Frankl.

22 Dyscalculia is a recognised problem associated with some parietal lobe lesions.

23 Parotid gland enlargement is associated with bulimia nervosa.

24 The Wernicke–Korsakoff syndrome is particularly associated with damage to the mamillary bodies.

25 Mothers in their first postnatal year are at the same risk of suicide as non-mothers of the same age.

---

21 True.
Paradoxical injunctions concern advice to the patient to act in a way that at first may seem to risk making the problem worse. Particular care is required in their use. A classic injunction is in the psychosexual therapy of Masters and Johnson (1970) where couples with sexual difficulties are told to avoid sex completely during the therapy. The prohibition serves only to heighten desire and reinforce the sexual act. Other injunctions might involve prescribing

symptoms, e.g. in patients with panic attacks, telling them to have four attacks a day (Frankl, 1970).

References:

- Frankl VE (ed.) (1970) *Psychotherapy and Existentialism: selected papers on logotherapy.* Souvenir Press, New York.
- Masters WH and Johnson VE (1970) *Human Sexual Inadequacy.* Churchill, London.

22 True.

Typically lesions of the parietal lobe may cause: constructional and dressing apraxia, sensory inattention, topographical agnosias, prosopagnosia, astereognosis, cortical sensory loss, dyscalculia, dysgraphia, finger agnosia, and right-left disorientation, among other symptoms and signs.

Reference:

- Lishman WA (1998) *Organic Psychiatry* (3e). Blackwell, London.

23 True.

Reference:

- Russell GFM (1979) Bulimia nervosa: an ominous variant of anorexia nervosa. *Br J Psychiatr.* **138:** 164.

24 True.

Wernicke's encephalopathy can involve damage to the walls of the third ventricle, periaqueductal region, floor of the fourth ventricle, some thalamic nuclei, paraventricular nuclei, mamillary bodies, brainstem and parts of the cerebellum. Only rarely can lesions be seen in the cerebral cortex.

25 False.

The standardised mortality ratio (ratio of deaths observed to deaths expected from age-specific death rates) for suicide by women in the first postnatal year indicates that the rate of suicide is only one-sixth of the expected rate, leading to the conclusion that child concerns are an important protective factor even in a high-risk population (Appleby, 1991).

Reference:

- Appleby L (1991) Suicide during pregnancy and in the first postnatal year. *BMJ.* **125:** 355–73.

---

26 Eventual suicide is more common among people who have previously left a suicide note during previous suicide attempts.

27 Causes of male erectile disorder include antihypertensives such as
atenolol.

28 Tourette's syndrome is associated with coprophagia.

29 Recognised features of Alzheimer-type dementia include prosopagnosia.

30 Recognised types of rating scales include Likert scales.

---

26 **True.**
Suicide notes among 'attempters' signal those at higher risk of eventual
suicide.

References:

- Dorpat T and Ripley H (1967) The relationship between attempted suicide and
committed suicide. *Compr Psychiatr*. **8**: 74–9.
- Tuckman J and Youngman W (1968) A scale for assessing suicide risk of
attempted suicides. *J Clin Psychol*. **24**: 17–19.

27 **True.**
Beta-blockers are associated with sexual dysfunction, but attendees at heart
clinics may have expectations about beta-blockers based on previous knowledge and this may affect their capacity to perform, so there may be a
psychological element to any sexual dysfunction.

References:

- Segraves RT (2003) Pharmacologic management of sexual dysfunction: benefits
and limitations. *CNS Spectrums*. **8**(3): 225–9.
- Silvestri A, Galetta P, Cerquetani E, Marazzi G, Patrizi R, Fini M and Rosano
GM (2003) Report of erectile dysfunction after therapy with beta-blockers is
related to patient knowledge of side effects and is reversed by placebo. *European
Heart Journal*. **24**(21): 1928–32.

28 **False.**
Coprolalia is the sporadic, involuntary and inappropriate swearing seen in
some patients with Tourette's. Coprophagia is the eating of faeces.

References:

- Stern JS, Burza S and Robertson MM (2005) Gilles de la Tourette's syndrome
and its impact in the UK. *Postgraduate Medical Journal*. **81**(951): 12–19.

- Singer HS (2005) Tourette's syndrome: from behaviour to biology. *Lancet Neurology.* 4(3): 149–59.

29 True.
Prosopagnosia is the inability to recognise faces and is characteristic of parietal lobe dysfunction.

30 True.
Likert scales are interval rating scales where a line is drawn with anchor points and spaces in between.

---

31 Astasia-abasia can be described as a dissociative disorder.

32 A metallic or 'copper penny' taste can be a feature of temporal lobe epilepsy.

33 The thalamus has no connection with visual pathways.

34 Akataphasia is a disorder of thought in speech.

35 Cotard's syndrome is the delusion of being pregnant in males.

---

31 True.
Astasia-abasia is an example of a dissociative motor disorder (ICD-10, F44.4). It is the inability to stand or walk through defect of will. Other examples of dissociative motor disorders are the apparent loss of ability to move the whole or a part of a limb, psychogenic ataxia, psychogenic aphonia and psychogenic dysphonia.

Reference:

- World Health Organization (1992) *ICD-10 Clinical Descriptions and Diagnostic Guidelines.* WHO, Geneva.

32 True.

33 False.
The thalamus is connected to visual, auditory and somaesthetic pathways.

34 True.
Akataphasia was defined by Kraepelin (1919). It is a disorder in the expression of thought in speech.

35 False.
Cotard's syndrome is a form of depressive psychosis characterised by nihilistic and hypochondriacal delusions – for instance, Cotard described patients being asked their name and saying they had none, or where they were born

and saying they were not born, or asked if they have a headache and saying they have no head. The delusion of being pregnant or having obstetric symptoms in a male, often when their partner is pregnant, is called Couvade syndrome.

---

36 Anhedonia is the absence of a hedonistic lifestyle.

37 Features of frontal lobe dysfunction include nominal aphasia.

38 Bleuler identified thought withdrawal as a primary symptom complex in schizophrenia.

39 Episodic anxiety is associated with mitral stenosis.

40 According to Fish (1967), dysmegalopsia is a sensory distortion.

---

36 False.
Anhedonia is the total lack of enjoyment in life or a 'loss of ability to experience pleasure'. It is a frequent characteristic of depression.

Reference:

- Snaith RP (1993) Anhedonia: a neglected symptom of psychopathology. *Psychological Medicine.* **23**: 957–66.

37 False.
In nominal aphasia the patient has difficulty recalling or recognising names of objects or other things which the patient should know well. The patient speaks fluently and grammatically and appears to have normal comprehension. The problem is often related to temporal or parietal lesions.

38 False.
It was Carl Schneider who identified the complex of thought withdrawal (*Gedankenentzug*) as a key symptom-complex in schizophrenia. This broad complex as defined by him included thought blocking, thought withdrawal, perplexity, thought insertion, passivity experiences and verbal derailment. The other two complexes he identified were the complex of inconsequence (*Sprunghaftigkeit*) and the complex of scattered thinking (*Faseln*).

Reference:

- Schneider C (1942) *Die Schizophrenen Symptomverbande.* Berlin.

39 True.
Mitral valve prolapse has been reported in a significant minority of patients with anxiety disorder but so has mitral stenosis.

References:

- Lichodziejewska B, Klos J, Rezler J, Grudzka K, Dluzniewska M, Budaj A and Ceremuzynski L (1997) Clinical symptoms of mitral valve prolapse are related to hypomagnesemia and attenuated by magnesium supplementation. *American Journal of Cardiology.* **79**(6): 768–72.
- Shuldham C, Goodman H, Fleming S, Tattersall K and Pryse-Hawkins H (2001) Anxiety, depression and functional capacity in older women with mitral valve stenosis. *International Journal of Nursing Practice.* 7(5): 322–8.

40 **True.**
Dysmegalopsia is a sensory distortion involving a change in spatial form, and may occur in retinal disease, disorders of accommodation, and temporal lobe lesions.

Reference:

- Fish F (1967) *Clinical Psychopathology.* Wright, Bristol.

---

41 Nicotinic acid deficiency is a cause of neuropathy.

42 Huntington's disease has incomplete penetrance in hereditary terms.

43 Chlorpromazine is routinely given intramuscularly and intravenously.

44 Temporal lobe dysfunction is associated with auditory agnosia.

45 An example of a third-person auditory hallucination would include: 'a voice inside my head saying: he's useless'.

---

41 **True.**
Nicotinic acid deficiency causes diarrhoea, polyneuropathy, glossitis, a dark, scaly dermatitis and sometimes a mild dementia.

42 **False.**
Huntington's disease was first described in 1872 and has latterly has been localised to chromosome 4. It has complete penetrance in hereditary terms.

43 **False.**
Intravenous chlorpromazine carries a very high risk of arrhythmia.

44 **True.**

45 **False.**
A hallucination is usually experienced in external space and this is experienced 'inside my head'.

46 A patient who says 'The voice says: go and jump. Jump now' may be experiencing a command hallucination.

47 A patient who says 'My wife and I often hear our next-door neighbours discussing us' is probably experiencing third-person auditory hallucinations.

48 Dosulepin may induce hallucinations.

49 Partially reversible causes of dementia include Wilson's disease.

50 Tremor may be a long-term side effect of lithium, independent of serum concentration.

46 **True.**

47 **False.**
The patient indicates that his wife can also hear the neighbours, suggesting this may be a real rather than a hallucinatory experience.

48 **True.**
Dosulepin may induce hallucinatory experiences by virtue of its cholinergic activity.

49 **True.**

50 **True.**
Long-term effects, independent of the serum concentration, include thirst, polyuria, tremor, weight gain (partially due to water retention), diarrhoea, and hypothyroidism.

51 The psychological defence mechanism of denial typically occurs in *normal* grief reactions.

52 Causes of delirium include rifampicin and isoniazid at therapeutic doses.

53 Depersonalisation frequently occurs in mania.

54 In a phobic disorder fear is out of proportion to the demands of the situation.

55 Poor insight is associated with poor performance on the Wisconsin Card Sorting Test.

51 **True.**

Reference:

● Rycroft C (1968) *A Critical Dictionary of Psychoanalysis*. Nelson, London.

52 **True.**
Various drugs at therapeutic doses can induce delirium in susceptible individuals, including among others: rifampicin and isoniazid (used in tuberculosis), codeine, benzodiazepines, antihistamines, methyldopa, ACE (angiotensin-converting enzyme) inhibitors, calcium channel blockers, indomethacin, ranitidine and cimetidine, steroids, tricyclic antidepressants, and various neuroleptics.

Reference:

● Bauer MS (2003) *Field Guide to Psychiatric Assessment and Treatment*. Lippincott, Williams and Wilkins, Philadelphia.

53 **False.**
Depersonalisation is recognised as occurring in bipolar affective disorder, but only in the depressive phase.

Reference:

● Sims A (2003) *Symptoms in the Mind*. Saunders, London.

54 **True.**
Marks (1969) listed four criteria for a phobia: fear is out of proportion to the demands of the situation, the phobia cannot be explained or reasoned away, it is not under voluntary control and the fear leads to avoidance behaviour.

Reference:

● Marks IM (1969) *Fears and Phobia*. Heinemann, London.

55 **True.**
Studies link poor insight with poor performance on the Wisconsin Card Sorting Test, perhaps suggesting a link with frontal lobe dysfunction.

Reference:

● Sims A (2003) *Symptoms in the Mind*. Saunders, London.

---

56 Weight gain is a frequent adverse effect associated with lithium use.

57 Seizures triggered by psychotropic drugs are a dose-independent adverse effect.

58 Males with post-traumatic stress disorder (PTSD) are significantly more likely to suffer with irritability than females with PTSD.

59 People with a high internal locus of control attribute success or failure to outside forces.

60 A fundamental attribution error occurs when an observer wrongly infers that an action has to do with internal traits rather than the environment.

---

56 **True.**
Weight gain is often associated with lithium use, possibly related to increased leptin levels. Leptin is an adipocyte hormone, regulating food intake and energy balance providing the hypothalamus with information on the amount of body fat.

Reference:

● Atmaca M, Kuloglu M, Tezcan E and Ustundag B (2002) Weight gain and serum leptin levels in patients on lithium treatment. *Neuropsychobiology.* **46**(2): 67–9.

57 **False.**
Seizures triggered by psychotropic drugs are a dose-dependent adverse effect. Among antipsychotics the most likely to induce seizures are chlorpromazine and clozapine. Among antidepressants the most likely to induce seizures are maprotiline and clomipramine.

Reference:

● Pisani F, Oteri G, Costa C, Di Raimondo G and Di Perri R (2002) Effects of psychotropic drugs on seizure threshold. *Drug Safety.* **25**(2): 91–110.

58 **True.**
Men with PTSD are significantly more likely than women with PTSD to suffer with irritability (p<0.05) and to use alcohol to excess (p<0.05).

Reference:

● Green B (2003) Post-traumatic stress disorder: symptom profiles in men and women. *Current Medical Research and Opinion.* **19**(3): 200–4.

59 **False.**
People with a high internal locus of control view themselves as having control over their own destinies.

60 **True.**

---

61 Operant conditioning involves reinforcement, which occurs whether or not certain behaviours occur.

62 According to Julian Rotter, expectancy is our belief that if we behave in a certain way this will predict our rewards.

63 The Sixteen Personality Factor Test (16PF) was developed by Carl Jung.

64 At the lowest level of Maslow's hierarchy of needs we find love and belongingness needs.

65 Learned helplessness is a concept researched on animals by psychologists using inescapable electric shocks on dogs.

---

61 **False.**
Operant conditioning involves reinforcement contingent upon a certain behaviour or set of behaviours.

62 **True.**
Julian Rotter developed social learning psychology and was responsible for notions such as internal and external locus of control. Essentially Rotter developed an idea that your reactions to the environment are based on your personal view of the world – i.e. your behaviours depend on your cognitions about the environment. Expectancy is our belief that if we behave in a certain way this will predictably lead to certain rewards.

Reference:

- Schultz SE and Schultz D (2004) *Theories of Personality* (8e). Wadsworth, Belmont.

63 **False.**
The Sixteen Personality Factor Test (16PF) was developed by Raymond Cattell.

64 **False.**
At the lowest level of Abraham Maslow's hierarchy of needs we find physiological needs; at the highest level we find self-actualisation.

65 True.
Psychologist Martin Seligman tested out his theory of learned helplessness in the 1970s by developing a series of experiments that gave dogs electric shocks in differing scenarios. Seligman found that prior exposure only to inescapable shock interfered with their ability to learn in a subsequent situation where avoidance or escape was indeed possible. Seligman used the term 'learned helplessness' to describe this phenomenon and argued that human depression had similar qualities.

Reference:

● Seligman ME (1992) *Helplessness – On Depression, Development and Death.* Freeman, New York.

---

66 Neurological soft signs are found more often in children at genetic risk of schizophreniform illness.

67 Neurological soft signs in schizophrenia are correlated with a loss of grey matter.

68 There is virtually no first-pass metabolism with clozapine.

69 Carbamazepine acts to increase the plasma level of risperidone.

70 Haloperidol is metabolised by the CYP1A2 system.

---

66 True.
The Helsinki High-Risk Study monitored women treated for schizophrenia-spectrum disorders in Helsinki mental hospitals before 1975, their offspring, and controls. They compared the development of high-risk and control group children, and investigated which factors predicted future psychiatric disorders. Compared with controls, children in the high-risk group had more emotional symptoms before school age, attentional problems and social inhibition at school age, and neurological soft signs throughout.

Reference:

● Niemi LT, Suvisaari JM, Haukka JK and Lonnqvist JK (2005) Childhood predictors of future psychiatric morbidity in offspring of mothers with psychotic disorder: results from the Helsinki High-Risk Study. *British Journal of Psychiatry.* **186:** 108–14.

67 True.
Higher rates of soft neurological signs (both motor and sensory) are associated with a reduction of grey matter volume of subcortical structures (putamen, globus pallidus and thalamus).

Reference:

- Dazzan P, Morgan KD, Orr KG, Hutchinson G, Chitnis X, Suckling J, Fearon P, Salvo J, McGuire PK, Mallett RM, Jones PB, Leff J and Murray RM (2004) The structural brain correlates of neurological soft signs in AESOP first-episode psychoses study. *Brain.* **127**(Pt 1): 143–53.

68 **False.**
There is an extensive first-pass metabolism with clozapine and only 27–50% of the dose reaches the systemic circulation unchanged.

Reference:

- Green B (2004) *Focus on Antipsychotics.* Petroc Press, Newbury.

69 **False.**
Carbamazepine acts to reduce the plasma level of risperidone by inducing hepatic enzymes. Some other drugs such as fluoxetine and tricyclic anti-depressants may increase the plasma level of risperidone.

70 **True.**

---

71 First-rank symptoms of schizophrenia include the conviction that someone else is moving one's limbs.

72 Dissocial personality disorder is frequently preceded by a diagnosis of conduct disorder.

73 A stereotyped pattern of drinking is an essential element in the alcohol-dependence syndrome as described by Edwards and Gross (1976).

74 Features of anorexia nervosa as described in ICD-10 include weight loss to 25% below expected weight.

75 A pioneer of word association testing was Carl Gustav Jung.

---

71 **True.**
First-rank symptoms of schizophrenia include hearing one's thoughts spoken aloud, hallucinatory conversations about the patient, a running commentary on thoughts and actions, bodily hallucinations attributed to third parties, thought withdrawal, thought insertion and other influences on thought, thought broadcasting, delusional perception, and passivity phenomena. Second-rank features include catatonic behaviour, secondary delusions and hallucinations other than those described above.

References:

- Jaspers K (1963) *General Psychopathology.* Manchester University Press, Manchester.
- Schneider K (1959) *Clinical Psychopathology.* Grune and Stratton, New York.

72 **True.**

73 **True.**
Edwards and Gross (1976) described the alcohol-dependence syndrome, which comprised a stereotyped pattern of drinking, prominence of alcohol-seeking behaviour, increased alcohol tolerance, repeated withdrawal symptoms, relief or avoidance of withdrawal by further drinking, a subjective awareness of a compulsion to drink, and relapse or re-instatement of drinking behaviour after abstinence.

Reference:

- Edwards G and Gross MM (1976) Alcohol dependence: provisional description of a clinical syndrome. *BMJ.* 1: 1058.

74 **True.**
Features of anorexia nervosa as described in ICD-10 include body weight at least 15% below that expected or Quetelet's body mass index being 17.5 or less. Quetelet's body mass index is the weight in kilograms divided by the square of the height in metres. Other features include a dread of fatness amounting to an overvalued idea, body-image distortion, self-induced weight loss, vomiting, purging, excessive exercise, use of appetite suppressants or diuretics, amenorrhoea in women and loss of sexual interest/potency in men, raised growth hormone and cortisol, changes in thyroid hormone metabolism and abnormal insulin secretion.

75 **True.**
Jung wrote some of the earliest papers on word association.

---

76 Catalepsy is a frequent side effect of clozapine.

77 High prolactin levels are a frequent problem with quetiapine.

78 According to Sigmund Freud, dreams often involve a latent content.

79 Temporal lobe dysfunction is associated with homonymous hemianopia.

80 Using purely open-ended questions in an interview virtually guarantees that all relevant clinical information is elicited.

76 **False.**
Clozapine is an atypical antipsychotic and does not induce catalepsy.

77 **False.**
Compared to placebo, quetiapine does not raise prolactin levels.

Reference:

● Green B (2004) *Focus on Antipsychotics*. Petroc Press, Newbury.

78 **True.**
The manifest content of a dream is that which is remembered and reported. The latent content involves the underlying memories, thoughts, fantasies and desires. The translation of the latent content into the manifest content is the dream work.

Reference:

● Freud S (1900) The interpretation of dreams. In: J Strachey (ed.) *Complete Psychological Works*, Vol. V. Hogarth Press, London.

79 **True.**

80 **False.**
Exclusively open-ended questioning does not guarantee gathering all the relevant clinical information in an interview mainly because non-professionals do not think like diagnosticians. High-sensitivity questions should be used to screen for specific psychiatric disorders and high-specificity questions to confirm or rule out the suspected diagnosis.

Reference:

● Bauer MS (2003) *A Field Guide to Psychiatric Assessment and Treatment.* Lippincott, Wiliams and Wilkins, New York.

---

81 Poverty of thought is associated with frontal lobe disorder.

82 The Beck Depression Inventory involves the use of a structured interview.

83 Papilloedema on neurological examination could signal severe anaemia.

84 Dysphonia is a defect of speech articulation.

85 Reduced libido is a feature of depression but not of post-traumatic stress disorder.

81 **True.**
Slowing of thought and motor activity are related to dorsolateral frontal lobe damage.

82 **False.**
The Beck Depression Inventory involves the use of a patient-completed questionnaire.

83 **True.**
There are numerous causes of papilloedema including severe anaemia, space-occupying lesions, meningitis, cerebral oedema, and lead poisoning to name but a few.

Reference:

- Malhi G, Matharu M and Hale A (2000) *Neurology for Psychiatrists*. Dunitz, London.

84 **False.**
Dysphonia is a defect of speech volume. Dysarthria is a defect of articulation with preserved language function.

85 **False.**
Reduced libido is a feature of both depression and PTSD.

---

86 Loneliness is an independent risk factor for depression in the elderly.

87 Narcissistic personality disorder is associated with inappropriate sexually seductive or provocative behaviour.

88 In Wilson's disease plaques of copper appear throughout the limbic system.

89 Postural hypotension is associated with paroxetine and chlorpromazine.

90 Unlike depressive disorder, dysthymic disorder is more common in men than women.

---

86 **True.**
Loneliness has been repeatedly shown to be a risk factor for old-age depression.

References:

- Adams KB, Sanders S and Auth EA (2004) Loneliness and depression in independent living retirement communities: risk and resilience factors. *Aging and Mental Health*. 8(6): 475–85.

- Green BH, Copeland JR, Dewey ME, Sharma V, Saunders PA, Davidson IA, Sullivan C and McWilliam C (1992) Risk factors for depression in elderly people: a prospective study. *Acta Psychiatrica Scandinavica*. 86(3): 213–17.

87 False.
'Inappropriate seductiveness in appearance or behaviour' is a criterion for F60.4 Histrionic Personality Disorder.

88 False.
Wilson's disease does not include *plaque* formation as such. Abnormal copper metabolism does result in deposition in various organs like the liver and brain. MRI scans show brain atrophy with hypodensities in thalamus and brainstem.

89 True.

90 False.
Dysthymic disorder is two to three times more common in women.

---

91 Factitious disorders involve patients simulating medical illness primarily for monetary gain.

92 Echopraxia often persists when the patient is asked to desist.

93 Late-onset depression is associated with subcortical neurological signs.

94 De Clerambault's syndrome is a variant of erotomania.

95 Delusions of infestation are only seen in depressive disorders.

---

91 False.
Factitious disorders involve patients simulating medical illness primarily to assume the sick role. Simulating symptoms for monetary gain or to avoid work would be an example of malingering or fraud.

92 True.
Echopraxia involves the patient mimicking the interviewer's movements and often persists after the interviewer has asked the patient to stop.

Reference:

- Sims A (2003) *Symptoms in the Mind*. Saunders, London.

93 True.
Comparisons of elderly people with and without late-onset depression find an excess of neurological signs in patients with depression, even after adjustment

for medication side effects. These included motor sequencing (dependent on intact frontal-striatal brain function), parkinsonian/subcortical features and primitive reflexes.

Reference:

● Baldwin R, Jeffries S, Jackson A, Sutcliffe C, Thacker N, Scott M and Burns A (2005) Neurological findings in late-onset depressive disorder: comparison of individuals with and without depression. *Br J Psychiatry.* **186**: 308–13.

94 True.
De Clerambault's syndrome is a variant of erotomania in which an individual, usually female, is deluded that a person of higher social status is in love with her. This person may have done nothing to deserve her attention and indeed may have no knowledge of her existence.

Reference:

● De Clerambault GG (1942) *Les psychoses passionelles. Oeuvre psychiatrique.* Presses Universitaire, Paris.

95 False.
Delusions of infestations can be seen in a variety of disorders, including affective disorders, schizophrenia and organic disorders with tactile hallucinations.

---

96 Hallucinations experienced only when there is an external stimulus are called extracampine hallucinations.

97 Psychotic symptoms in the general population are independently associated with cannabis use.

98 Depression, anxiety disorder, panic disorder and alcohol dependence are all more common in females than males.

99 Neuroticism in a person is more likely to lead to later psychopathology than in a 'normal' personality.

100 Lithium intoxication only occurs at high serum levels.

---

96 False.
Extracampine hallucinations are hallucinations experienced outside the possible field of awareness – for instance a patient hearing the voices of people talking about him in a distant house (without the use of technology such as a telephone!). When an external stimulus is needed to trigger a hallucination, e.g. a radio or TV triggering auditory hallucinations, then this is termed a functional hallucination.

97 **True.**
Research on the experience of psychotic symptoms in the general population found that about 5% have some psychotic symptomatology on self-report. There were independent associations with cannabis dependence, alcohol dependence, victimisation, recent stressful life events, lower intellectual ability and neurotic symptoms.

Reference:

- Johns LC, Cannon M, Singleton N, Murray RM, Farrell M, Brugha T, Bebbington P, Jenkins R and Meltzer H (2004) Prevalence and correlates of self reported psychotic symptoms in the British population. *Br J Psychiatry.* **185:** 298–305.

98 **False.**
Alcohol dependence is more often found in males than females.

99 **True.**
Neuroticism as conceptualised by Eysenck is identified as a significant personality trait and is a broad vulnerability factor for various comorbid psychiatric disorders.

Reference:

- Khan AA, Jacobson KC, Gardner CO, Prescott CA and Kendler KS (2005) Personality and comorbidity of common psychiatric disorders. *Br J Psychiatry.* **186:** 190–6.

100 **False.**
Lithium intoxication can occur at 'therapeutic' serum levels, although usually it is at higher levels. Early symptoms of mild toxicity include nausea, diarrhoea, blurred vision, polyuria, lightheadedness, fine resting tremor, muscle weakness and sleepiness. More serious levels of toxicity produce confusion, blackouts, twitches and choreoathetoid movements, convulsions, heart block and other dysrhythmias, and coma.

Reference:

- Haddad P, Dursun S and Deakin B (2004) *Adverse Syndromes and Psychiatric Drugs.* Oxford University Press, Oxford.

Extended Matching Items

> Q1 Cited risk factors for tardive dyskinesia include:
>
> - length of exposure to antipsychotics
> - alcohol consumption
> - male sex
> - negative symptoms of schizophrenia
> - previous head injury
> - diabetes mellitus
> - earlier drug-induced parkinsonism.

A1 Cited risk factors for tardive dyskinesia include:

- length of exposure to antipsychotics   T
- alcohol consumption   T
- male sex   F
- negative symptoms of schizophrenia   T
- previous head injury   T
- diabetes mellitus   T
- earlier drug-induced parkinsonism   T

Diabetes mellitus is associated with a 50% increase in risk. Female gender is a risk factor as are 'organic' brain dysfunction or damage, and early extra-pyramidal side effects.

References:

- Jeste DV and Caligiuri MP (1993) Tardive dyskinesia. *Schizophrenia Bulletin.* 19(2): 303–15.
- Woerner MG, Saltz BL, Kane JM, Lieberman JA and Alvir JM (1993) Diabetes and development of tardive dyskinesia. *American Journal of Psychiatry.* 150(6): 966–8.

> Q2 Lithium interacts adversely and significantly with:
>
> - ACE inhibitors
> - digoxin
> - fluoxetine
> - gabapentin
> - hypoglycaemics

- lamotrigine
- indomethacin
- phenytoin
- theophylline
- bendroflumethiazide
- warfarin.

A2 Lithium interacts adversely and significantly with:

- ACE inhibitors   T
- digoxin   F
- fluoxetine   T
- gabapentin   F
- hypoglycaemics   F
- lamotrigine   F
- indomethacin   T
- phenytoin   T
- theophylline   T
- bendroflumethiazide   T
- warfarin   F

Lithium interacts with ACE inhibitors to produce lithium toxicity especially in the elderly. Both gabapentin and lithium are excreted renally, but there is little interaction. Indomethacin and lithium interact such that there is a 60% increase in lithium levels. Lithium may be used to improve glucose metabolism and assist oral hypoglycaemics. Phenytoin and lithium produce lithium neurotoxicity. Theophylline reduces lithium levels by 20–30%. Bendroflumethiazide reduced lithium excretion by 24% or more.

References:

- Licht RW *et al.* Danish Psychiatric Association and the Child and Adolescent Psychiatric Association in Denmark (2003) Psychopharmacological treatment with lithium and antiepileptic drugs: suggested guidelines from the Danish Psychiatric Association and the Child and Adolescent Psychiatric Association in Denmark. *Acta Psychiatrica Scandinavica.* Supplementum. **419**: 1–22.
- Katona CL (2001) Psychotropics and drug interactions in the elderly patient. *International Journal of Geriatric Psychiatry.* **16** (suppl. 1): S86–90.
- Sayal KS, Duncan-McConnell DA, McConnell HW and Taylor DM (2000) Psychotropic interactions with warfarin. *Acta Psychiatrica Scandinavica.* **102**(4): 250–5.

Q3 The following may give rise to dementia in childhood:

A   Rett syndrome
B   Pelizaeus-Merzbacher disease
C   adrenoleukodystrophy
D   multiple sclerosis
E   metachromatic leukodystrophy
F   pervasive refusal syndrome
G   subacute sclerosing panencephalitis.

A3 The following may give rise to dementia in childhood:

A	Rett syndrome	T
B	Pelizaeus-Merzbacher disease	T
C	adrenoleukodystrophy	T
D	multiple sclerosis	T
E	metachromatic leukodystrophy	T
F	pervasive refusal syndrome	F
G	subacute sclerosing panencephalitis	T

There are over 600 possible causes of childhood dementia, all of which are rare. These may present to psychiatrists with depression or psychotic phenomenon. Most causes are irreversible.

Reference:

● Lask B, Taylor S and Nunn K (2003) *Practical Child Psychiatry. The clinician's guide.* BMJ Publishing Group, London.

Group Exercise: Risk Assessment

After a case conference or presentation, form a group and brainstorm with colleagues as to the potential risks posed by a clinical patient. The exercise is interesting sometimes because it highlights the strength (or lack of strength) of evidence for various quoted risks and how other risks are potentially ignored. The area of risk assessment is a crucial one and demonstrating a strategy for risk assessment in Clinicals (at Part I and Part II) and PMPs can demonstrate that you will be a potentially safe consultant colleague.

For the purpose of the exercise photocopy the Risk Assessment Matrix (RAM) on page 45 and try to fill it out for your chosen example patient. The matrix challenges you to evaluate the evidence for each risk and its level. Remember to treat the exercise seriously – respect the results and, as ever, ensure patient confidentiality is maintained.

Suggested reading:

- Gunn J (1993) Dangerousness. In: J Gunn and PJ Taylor (eds) *Forensic Psychiatry – clinical, legal and ethical issues*. Butterworth Heinemann, London, pp.587–98.
- Higgins N, Watts D, Bindman J, Slade M and Thornicroft G (2005) Assessing violence in general adult psychiatry. *Psychiatric Bulletin*. **29**: 131–3.
- Munro E and Rumgay J (2000) Role of risk assessment in reducing homicides in people with mental illness. *British Journal of Psychiatry*. **176**: 116–20.
- Szmukler G (2001) Violence risk prediction in practice. *British Journal of Psychiatry*. **178**: 84–5.
- Webster CD, Douglas KS, Eaves D and Hart SD (2001) *HCR 20. Assessing Risk for Violence*. Mental Health, Law and Policy Institute, Simon Fraser University, Vancouver.

Risk Assessment Matrix

This matrix was developed at Cheadle Royal Hospital for use on its PICUs (psychiatric intensive care units) by Dr Ben Green and Jenny Clarke. The advantage of the RAM is that it can be represented on one side of a piece of paper, while many more comprehensive risk assessment tools often 'lose' information within complicated formats. The RAM is intended to be used to develop care plans.

Please try and qualify each risk by indicating strength of evidence for this.

1 No known evidence
2 No evidence, but predicted from at-risk characteristics
3 Threatened in the past
4 Threatened during this episode of illness
5 Documented evidence prior to this episode
6 Documented evidence during this episode

Risk	PICU	Open ward	Community
Suicide			
Self-harming			
Sexually inappropriate assault			
Physical aggression			
Fire risk			
Absconding			
Substance misuse			
Self-neglect			
Poor compliance			
Poor insight			
Criminal activity			
Verbal hostility (e.g. racist)			
Exploitation (e.g. sexual)			
Other risk (e.g. arson)			

Source of evidence

Previous notes	
Social services	
Probation	
Patient	
Carer	
Police	
Current admission	

MRCPsych Part I: OSCE

Ben Green

The clinical examination in the Part I MRCPsych examination used to require candidates to travel to various hospitals around the country and interview a real patient, then present the case to two examiners. To test their interview technique the candidate would also be asked to question the patient in front of the examiners. The examination involved a degree of unpredictability, but perhaps did reflect real life in this regard and it also tested the candidate's ability to make sense of the whole of the patient's history and mental state examination and present this to the examiners.

The change from the patient history to an OSCE offers a possibility of standardisation in that, clinically, scenarios faced are controlled and repeated between candidates and, of course, actors can almost endlessly repeat a presentation, whereas real-life patients may fluctuate in terms of symptoms and signs. The actors are well-trained professionals and can simulate patients' symptoms and distress very well.

If a candidate does not pass the OSCE they must fail the entire Part I examination, no matter how well they have performed in the Written Paper.

The OSCE seeks to test the clinical and communication skills of psychiatrists and these are observed by a consultant psychiatrist examiner at every station. The actors may also provide feedback on how well, or badly, they think a candidate performs. The same actor/examiner combination will see numerous candidates performing in the same scenario and so they form a good idea of the range of abilities that candidates have.

The examiners are asked beforehand to screen photos of candidates to ensure that they do not know the candidates they will examine so that there is no conflict of interest.

The format of the OSCE

The OSCE is currently held in large venues that may accommodate four circuits simultaneously over three days. The venues are functional in nature and can be cavernous, cold and dispiriting. The ambience is one of a large-scale production line rather than anything else. Examiners and actors are bussed in from their hotels in the morning and bussed back at the end of what is a long and tiring day. The examiners and actors will be at the venue from 8.15 a.m. to 6.00 p.m. and this may produce the problem of fatigue.

Each circuit has 12 stations. A station may be a booth with a floor space of about four square metres, so space is restricted. Usually there will be just an examiner and actor in the booth, but sometimes there may be an observer (mainly to monitor the conduct of the exam – the scenario and the examiner) as well.

At each station the candidate is asked to perform a specific task. The task is attached to the wall outside each station and you will be expected to read this before going into the station and basically just get on with the task. *Read the task carefully.* The examiner checks the candidate name and number. The examiner may briefly introduce themselves for politeness' sake, but essentially *you* are expected to take control of the situation. There is another copy of the instructions inside the booth so you can refer to this again if you need to. You may notice the examiner watching you, and listening carefully to your questions' content and style, making notes. Only direct comments to the examiner if the instructions specifically tell you to. The examiners do not generally interrupt.

The task instructions may help you focus your efforts by advising you not to do certain things, e.g. in a neurological examination of the lower limbs to avoid dermatome examination of the sphincters. Other injunctions not to do something may be designed to spare the actor – for instance, an injunction not to do pain testing in a neurological examination.

Responding to the examiner's own criticism that there was a lack of inter-action between candidates and examiners in the exam design, the College has recently introduced some interaction. For instance, the candidate may be asked to role-play a telephone discussion with a consultant. An example is given below.

The scenarios are drawn from adult or old age psychiatry and would be appropriate to a junior trainee psychiatrist.

Skills tested according to the College are:

- history taking
- examination skills
- practical skills/use of equipment

- emergency management
- communication skills.

Candidates are told the circuit and the number of the station they are to begin at on entering the examination room.

Each station lasts seven minutes and begins with a bell or similar tone. After six minutes the bell rings again to warn the candidate that they have one minute left. When seven minutes are up the candidate must leave and go to the next station and wait outside (and read the next scenario). If the candidate finishes the task before the end of the seven minutes they should wait inside the booth, leaving at the end of seven minutes. Further conversation with the examiner or patient is not necessary.

The wait outside the booth is for one minute – only just enough time for the candidate to read the scenario and gather their thoughts about how to tackle it.

The candidate repeats the process until all the stations have been visited.

What are the examiners doing?

Each station has an individualised marksheet with specific objectives that the examiner must look out for. For instance, a station about a cardiological examination may ask the examiner to note whether the candidate examines for 'radial-radial delay'. No objective is left unmarked and there is only one grade for each objective. A global rating is present at the end of the marksheet, but earlier, specific objectives may have a crucial pass or fail role and may 'trump' the global rating. The examiner is not always aware of what the critical objective might be for a station.

Some information is given to examiners though. For instance, on a station where the candidate is asked to assess persecutory delusions and guilt the examiner may be told: 'This station tests the candidate's ability to assess the form and content of abnormal thoughts and explore how these abnormal ideas might have developed'. Objectives or skills that might be rated (each item attracting one mark) on the marksheet could include:

- communication skills
- nature (form and content) of beliefs
- evaluation of falseness of beliefs
- evaluation of conviction
- eliciting other abnormal phenomena
- global rating.

For the telephone conversation task (scenario 17) the examiner might be asked to rate you on your ability to describe mental capacity coherently and reason how this is applied to your assessment. The final decision as to whether the patient has or has not got mental capacity may not be so relevant as how you reason this.

The rating system for each objective would be on a five-point scale:

- A = Excellent
- B = Good
- C = Average
- D = Fail
- E = Severe Fail.

Examples of scenarios

As good practice the total number and type of scenarios will change over time, according to how well they discriminate between pass and fail candidates. The scenarios also change between sessions of the exam – that is, between morning and afternoon and between days. Asking candidates who have sat the morning session what their scenarios were will not give you any guide as to what the afternoon's scenarios will be. For instance, the physical examination station may be a cardiological examination in the morning and a neurological examination in the afternoon.

The following are typical scenarios and tasks:

1 *A 19-year-old man is found wandering the neighbourhood by police at 2 a.m. He is shouting at people who are not there. Interview him and establish what his experience is.*

2 *A 24-year-old girl is referred by her GP after a failure of counselling treatment for her eating disorders. Establish whether she has bulimia nervosa.*

3 *The surgical team have made a referral to the liaison psychiatry service. A patient with bowel carcinoma is refusing consent. He has had depression in the past. Establish whether he has the mental capacity to give or withhold consent.*

4 *The police have brought a 20-year-old student to the accident and emergency department. She has lacerated her wrists trying to get through a window to attack her half-brother because she thought he was trying to brainwash her. Explore her thoughts and experiences.*

5 *A 25-year-old woman, who has a boyfriend, has recently been started on lithium carbonate for bipolar affective disorder. Discuss the benefits and risks of lithium therapy with her.*

6 A 46-year-old man has a wrongly held belief that the police are looking for him in relation to a crime. He has gone to the police to give himself up. What is the nature of his belief?

7 A 40-year-old woman has a past history of anxiety and has recently developed episodes of anxiety with marked physical symptoms. Establish the nature of these episodes.

8 A patient's daughter has asked to see you about her mother's treatment with donepezil. Explain its mode of action and side effects.

9 A 76-year-old lady attends the accident and emergency department. She has been found wandering in the centre of town and according to police officers she is 'strange in manner'. The police have brought her to hospital. Assess her cognitive function.

10 A 70-year-old man has a history of dizziness, hemiparesis, 'confusion' and mood lability. Assess him physically.

11 You are asked to see an irate relative. Her son is being detained for assessment of third-person auditory hallucinations over recent months. Her son also has delusions about an alien 'lizard race'. His mother thinks this is all due to smoking cannabis and spending too much time on the internet. Try to address her concerns appropriately.

12 A man with bipolar affective disorder is transferred to your hospital, handcuffed and appropriately sedated with haloperidol. Establish a working diagnosis.

13 A middle-aged man with a history of panic attacks describes palpitations. Examine his cardiovascular system.

14 A middle-aged woman with a history of mood lability, disinhibition and severe headaches is now complaining of visual disturbances. Assess her visual fields and perform a fundoscopy.

15 You are asked to see the mother of a young man with treatment-resistant schizophrenia. He has been on numerous different combinations of drugs in the past and the team have decided that clozapine should be prescribed now. The patient has consented for you to talk to his mother about the benefits and side effects of clozapine.

16 *You are asked to assess a 53-year-old man who has been found to have ECG changes suggestive of a heart attack. The cardiology SHO is worried because the man is refusing to stay in hospital. He has a past history of depressive psychosis. Can he be compulsorily admitted? Assess his mental capacity and any need for detention.*

17 *Regarding the 53-year-old patient you have just assessed in the previous scenario, please now discuss this on the telephone with the on-call consultant, presenting your assessment and reasoning whether the patient can or should be detained.*

18 *A 75-year-old widow who lives alone has been admitted compulsorily for assessment. She has ideas that her neighbours are plotting against her to kill her and she suffers with hallucinations. Assess her perceptual abnormalities and thought content. Do not assess her cognition or attempt a risk assessment.*

19 *A woman is brought into the hospital by a friend who noted that she had not turned up for work. She has been low in mood in recent weeks. Over the weekend she has been building a funeral pyre in the back garden as she says she is dead and needs to be cremated. Explore her mood and beliefs.*

20 *A young woman has been admitted complaining of loss of sensation in her legs and abdomen and an inability to walk. She has not lost bowel or bladder control. Perform a limited neurological examination of her lower limbs. Note: pinprick/pain sensation should not be tested. You should not examine dermatomes associated with sphincters.*

Hints

Ensure you respect the patient's dignity – for instance, in uncovering an actor during the physical examination ask permission (but also ensure that you do adequately expose an area for examination). It can get quite cold for actors being repeatedly uncovered for most of the morning so please make sure you give them their blankets back...

   If you are given a specific task (e.g. explaining the mode of action and side effects of treatment with clozapine, donepezil or lithium) focus on this and do not spend too much time gathering historical information. Some information gathering would seem germane (e.g. establishing whether a young woman on lithium uses contraception), but too much will lead you to run out of time for quite specific things that you are being marked for. For instance, in explaining treatments, you may need to take control of the conversation (without appearing brusque), give information and check understanding. Try and match the level of the information you give according to the level of understanding (without erring too much towards being patronising). Avoid medical jargon or specialised terms that can be just as easily described in plain English.

Demonstrate that you are 'safe' by asking questions (where relevant) about suicidal ideation/plans and dangerousness.

Summarise what the patient has told you occasionally or use clarifying statements in your interview style so that the examiner knows what you are thinking of the patient's symptoms.

Be sure to practise detailed examinations of various body systems until they are really slick. Ask medical SpRs (specialist registrars) or consultants if they can watch your technique and give advice. Candidates who are unfamiliar with physical examination techniques or who perform them in an unorthodox manner or illogical order tend to stand out from the crowd.

Focus yourself: some scenarios have quite a few aspects to them – what are the key aspects you should address? The wording of the scenario will suggest what the objectives of the station are.

Use a standardised questioning style – such as that in the SCAN/Present State Examination (based on work from Wing *et al.*, 1974) – or suggested questions in good books on psychiatric interviewing, e.g. *The First Interview: revised for DSM-IV* by James Morrison or *Psychiatric Interviewing* by Shawn Christopher Shea (1998). Poorly phrased questions give a bad impression and often do not elicit the necessary symptoms/signs.

Use video of any practice interviewing sessions with other colleagues – what feedback can you give yourself on presentation and your style of questioning?

The examiners are meant to write quite detailed notes on the marksheets should you fail a station. As these represent data on file about you, you may be legally entitled to see copies of these and these may give valuable feedback for future performance.

Group Exercise: OSCE

1   Work with two other colleagues for this exercise. This involves three role-plays, with each one of you eventually playing all three roles. The three roles are doctor, patient and examiner.
2   Choose one of the scenarios from above and work through a seven-minute role-play.
3   The examiner should watch the doctor's interview of the patient and then feed back to the doctor what they thought was good about the interview and suggestions for improvement. By the end of the three role-plays you

should all have a pretty good idea of how best to approach such a scenario in the OSCE.

Further reading

- Morrison J (1995) *The First Interview: revised for DSM-IV*. Guilford Press, London.
- Shea SC (1998) *Psychiatric Interviewing: the art of understanding* (2e). Saunders, Philadelphia.
- Sommers-Flanagan J and Sommers-Flanagan R (2002) *Clinical Interviewing*. John Wiley and Sons Inc, New York.
- Wing JK, Cooper JE and Sartorius N (1974) *The Measurement and Classification of Psychiatric Symptoms*. Cambridge University Press, London.
- Wing JK, Nixon JM, Mann SA and Leff JP (1977) Reliability of the PSE (ninth edition) used in a population study. *Psychol Med.* 7: 505–16.
- Wing JK, Sartorius N and Ustun TB (1998) *Diagnosis and Clinical Measurement in Psychiatry: reference manual for SCAN/PSE-10*. Cambridge University Press, Cambridge.

MRCPsych Part II: Basic Sciences Written Paper

Individual Statements

---

1   The majority of cases of frontotemporal dementia demonstrate Pick-type histological changes.

2   Alzheimer-type senile plaques are commonly found in the brains of patients with Dementia with Lewy Bodies.

3   In cerebrovascular disease incomplete infarcts are mainly due to hypoperfusion.

4   In contrast to young-onset schizophrenia, computed tomography (CT) and magnetic resonance imaging (MRI) studies of late-onset schizophrenia generally report a reduced ventricular to brain ratio compared to age-matched healthy controls due to increased cerebral atrophy in late-onset schizophrenia.

5   The neurofibrillary tangles in Alzheimer's disease contain paired helical filaments of hyperphosphorylated tau protein.

---

1   **False.**

The minority show Pick-type changes, hence the term frontotemporal dementia is preferred to Pick's disease.

Reference:

● Snowden J, Neary D and Mann DMA (2002) Frontotemporal dementia. *British Journal of Psychiatry*. **180**: 140–3.

2   **True.**
The other characteristic pathological change of Alzheimer's disease – neurofibrillary tangles – are few in the brains of Dementia with Lewy Bodies.

Reference:

● Weiner MF (1999) Dementia associated with Lewy bodies. *Archives of Neurology.* **56**: 1441–2.

3   **True.**
Complete infarcts are mainly caused by vascular occlusion and incomplete infarcts by hypoperfusion.

Reference:

● Brun A (2003) Vascular burden of the white matter. *International Psychogeriatrics.* **15**(Suppl. 1): 53–8. (This supplement completely covers the vascular burden of the brain and dementia.)

Also a good text:

● Chui E, Gustafson L, Ames D and Folstein MF (eds) (2000) *Cerebrovascular Disease and Dementia; pathology, neuropsychiatry and management.* Martin Dunitz, London.

4   **False.**
The general neuroimaging finding is increased ventricular to brain ratio, similar to young-onset schizophrenia, due to ventricular dilatation. There is no increase in cerebral atrophy.

Reference:

● Howard R *et al.* (2000) Late onset and very late onset schizophrenia like psychosis: an international consensus. *American Journal of Psychiatry.* **157**: 172–8.

5   **True.**

Reference:
Many texts describe the neuropathology of Alzheimer's disease, e.g.

● Anderton BH (1999) Molecular biology of Alzheimer's disease. In: R Howard (ed.) *Everything You Need to Know About Old Age Psychiatry.* Wrightson Biomedical Publishing Ltd, London, pp.3–16.

6 Use of the atypical antipsychotic risperidone in dementia is associated with an increased risk of cerebral ischaemic events.

7 Memantine is a drug treatment for moderate and severe Alzheimer's
disease that has its effects by inhibiting the enzyme butyryl cholinesterase.

8 PCP is an NMDA glutamate receptor agonist.

9 The mean hereditability of ADHD is 0.75 which means about 25%
of the aetiologic contribution is genetic.

10 DRD3 and COMT are putative genes predisposing to schizophrenia.

6   **True.**
Randomised clinical trial data suggests a threefold increased risk for
risperidone and twofold risk for olanzapine.

Reference:
www.mca.gov.uk/aboutagency/regframework/csm/csmframe.htm

7   **False.**
Memantine is a drug treatment for moderate and severe Alzheimer's disease
but is a non-competitive N methyl D aspartate (NMDA) receptor antagonist
believed to have effect by regulating the excitatory neurotransmitter glutamate.

Reference:

- Mobius HJ (2003) Memantine: update on the current evidence. *International
  Journal of Geriatric Psychiatry.* **18**(supplement 1): S47–54. (This whole supplement is devoted to memantine, glutamatergic neurotransmission and Alzheimer's
  disease.)

8   **False.**
PCP (phencyclidine) is an NMDA glutamate receptor antagonist, which
explains, to some extent, its psychotomimetic effects.

9   **False.**
The mean hereditability of ADHD (attention deficit hyperactivity disorder) is
0.75 which means about 75% of the aetiologic contribution is genetic.

Reference:

- Thapar A, Holmes, J, Poulton K *et al.* (1999) Genetic basis of attention deficit
  and hyperactivity. *Br J Psych.* **179**: 105–11.

10 True.

Different studies have replicated evidence for a few candidate genes that increase susceptibility to schizophrenia, including DRD3 and COMT.

References:

- Park TW, Yoon KS, Kim JH, Park WY, Hirvonen A and Kang D (2002) Functional catechol-O-methyltransferase gene polymorphism and susceptibility to schizophrenia. *European Neuropsychopharmacology.* **12**(4): 299–303.
- Waterwort DM, Bassett AS and Brzustowicz LM (2002) Recent advances in the genetics of schizophrenia. *Cellular and Molecular Life Sciences.* **59**(2): 331–48.

---

11 Lifetime prevalence of major depressive disorder is about 5%.

12 Women are equally likely as men to suffer anxiety and mood disorders in any 12-month period.

13 The prevalence of ADHD in adults is less than 0.1%.

14 Most patients with schizophrenia do not have a relative with schizophrenia.

15 The Clock Drawing Test is a measure of parietal lobe function.

---

11 False.

The European Study of the Epidemiology of Mental Disorders (ESEMeD) found a lifetime prevalence for major depressive disorder of 12.8%.

Reference:

- ESEMeD/MHEDEA 2000 Investigators (2004) Prevalence of mental disorders in Europe. *Acta Psychiatrica Scandinavica.* **104**(suppl. 420): 21–7.

12 False.

The European Study of the Epidemiology of Mental Disorders (ESEMeD) found that the 12-month prevalence of anxiety and mood disorders in women was twice that of men.

Reference:

- ESEMeD/MHEDEA 2000 Investigators (2004) Prevalence of mental disorders in Europe. *Acta Psychiatrica Scandinavica.* **104**(suppl. 420): 21–7.

13 False.

The prevalence of ADHD in adults in the US is quoted as between 1% and 6%.

Reference:

- Wender PH, Wolf LE and Wanestein J (2001) Adults with ADHD: an overview. *Ann NY Acad Sci.* **931**: 1–16.

14 **True.**

15 **False.**
The Clock Drawing Test is a cognitive screening instrument like the Mini Mental State Examination.

Reference:

- Shulman KI (2000) Clock-drawing: is it the ideal cognitive screening test? *International Journal of Geriatric Psychiatry.* **15**: 548–61.

---

16 There is overlap between putative susceptibility genes for bipolar affective disorder and schizophrenia.

17 The COMT gene lies on chromosome 6 and is a putative susceptibility gene for schizophrenia.

18 Research studies suggest that approximately 5% of children are experiencing a psychiatric disorder at any one time.

19 Bandura developed the conception of reciprocal determinism.

20 The zone of proximal development (ZPD) was a concept developed by Rousseau.

---

16 **True.**
There is some overlap between possible susceptibility genes for bipolar affective disorder and schizophrenia (Berrettini, 2000). Such genes include COMT (Harrison and Weinberger, 2004) and G72/G30 (Hattori *et al.*, 2003; Chen *et al.*, 2004; Chumakov *et al.*, 2002).

References:

- Berrettini WH (2000) Are schizophrenia and bipolar disorders related? *Biol Psychiatry.* **48**: 531–38.
- Chen YS *et al.* (2004) Association between bipolar affective disorder and G72/G30. *Mol Psychiatry.* **9**: 87–92.
- Chumakov I *et al.* (2002) *Proc Natl Acad Sci USA.* **99**: 13675–80.
- Harrison and Weinberger (2004) *Mol Psychiatry.* Epub, 20 July.
- Hattori E *et al.* (2003) Polymorphisms at the G72/G30 locus. *Am J Hum Genet.* **72**: 1131–40.

17 **False.**
The COMT gene is a putative susceptibility gene for schizophrenia (Harrison and Weinberger, 2004). However, it lies on the long arm of chromosome 22 (22q11) near the chromosomal area deleted in velocardiofacial syndrome.

References:

● Harrison and Weinberger (2004) *Mol Psychiatry*. Epub, 20 July.

18 **False.**
Most studies suggest figures ranging from 10% to 20%.

Reference:

● Rutter M, Hersov L and Taylor E (1995) *Child and Adolescent Psychiatry: modern approaches*. Blackwell Science, Oxford.

19 **True.**
This involves behaviour, personal factors (cognitions, affect and biological events) and environmental influences all interacting together.

Reference:

● Bandura A (1986) *Social Foundations of Thought and Action: a social-cognitive theory*. Prentice-Hall, Englewood Cliffs.

20 **False.**
The zone of proximal development (ZPD) was described by Vygotsky to describe the 'gap' between what individuals can achieve alone and what they can achieve with the help of a more knowledgeable person.

---

21 Poor adolescent cognitive performance predicts later development of schizophrenia.

22 Disturbance of attention and awareness during delirium is related to dysfunction of the anterior cingulate cortex.

23 The prevalence of alcoholism in women is not affected by sexual preference.

24 Evidence suggests cognitive behavioural therapy (CBT) is ineffective in amphetamine abuse.

25 Visuospatial working memory and verbal working memory are impaired in MDMA ('ecstasy') users.

21 **True.**
The main known risk factors in the development of schizophrenia are genetic factors, pregnancy and delivery complications, slow neuromotor development, and deviant cognitive and academic performance. However, their effect size and predictive power are small. Developmental precursors such as poor cognitive premorbid performance are not necessarily specific to schizophrenia, but also common to other psychotic disorders.

Reference:

● Isohanni M *et al.* (2004) Developmental precursors of psychosis. *Current Psychiatry Reports.* **6**(3): 168–75.

22 **True.**
Functional neuroimaging studies in humans have provided evidence that a frontal network including the anterior cingulate cortex (ACC) plays an important role in attention and awareness.

Reference:

● Reischies FM, Neuhaus AH and Hansen ML (2005) Electrophysiological and neuropsychological analysis of a delirious state: the role of the anterior cingulate gyrus. *Psychiatry Research.* **138**(2): 171–81.

23 **False.**
Although sexual preference in men (heterosexual/bisexual/homosexual) does not appear to affect rates of alcoholism, homosexuality and bisexuality in women appear to be associated with significantly higher rates of alcohol consumption.

Reference:

● Drabble L, Midanik LT and Trocki K (2005) Reports of alcohol consumption and alcohol-related problems among homosexual, bisexual and heterosexual respondents: results from the 2000 National Alcohol Survey. *Journal of Studies on Alcohol.* **66**(1): 111–20.

24 **False.**
A relatively few sessions of CBT have been shown to be associated with significantly better rates of abstinence in regular amphetamine users.

Reference:

● Baker A, Lee NK, Claire M, Lewin TJ *et al.* (2005) Brief cognitive behavioural interventions for regular amphetamine users: a step in the right direction. *Addiction.* **100**(3): 367–78.

25 **True.**
Verbal and visuospatial working memory and other executive deficits have been observed in ecstasy users.

Reference:

• Wareing M, Fisk JE, Murphy P *et al.* (2005) Visuo-spatial working memory deficits in current and former users of MDMA ('ecstasy'). *Human Psychopharmacology.* 20(2): 115–23.

---

26 The thalamus has no connection with spinal tracts.

27 Friedreich's ataxia mainly affects the anterior spinal tracts.

28 The cingulate gyrus is part of the so-called limbic system.

29 Causes of neuropathy include systemic lupus erythematosus (SLE).

30 Acute intermittent porphyria is secondary to reduced protoporphyrinogen oxidase activity.

---

26 **False.**
The thalamus does have connections with spinal tracts: perhaps the best known reticular pathways include the lateral and anterior spinothalamic tracts.

27 **False.**
Friedreich's ataxia has an early onset, between 5 and 15 years. The ataxia is secondary to a degeneration of the posterior columns and lateral columns, especially the corticospinal and posterior spinocerebellar tracts. The heart muscle becomes thickened and fibrosed leading to death in the fifth decade of life from cardiac failure. Recognised features include ataxia, upper limb incoordination, nystagmus, intention tremor, dysarthria, extensor plantar reflexes, poor proprioception, pes cavus, scoliosus, and optic atrophy.

28 **True.**
The limbic system regulates the hypothalamus and is important for emotional and affective functions, and the control of motivation and actions. It incorporates the olfactory bulbs and lobes, hippocampus, amygdala, cingulate cortex, the septal area, fornix, hippocampus and parahippocampal gyrus.

29 **True.**
Severe neurological involvement in systemic lupus erythematosus (NPSLE) is one of the most dreadful complications of the disease. IV cyclophosphamide and IV methylprednisolone are sometimes used for neurological complications. The exact pathology behind the neuropathy is yet to be confirmed.

References:

• Barile-Fabris L, Ariza-Andraca R, Olguin-Ortega L, Jara LJ, Fraga-Mouret A, Miranda-Limon JM, Fuentes de la Mata J, Clark P, Vargas F and Alocer-Varela J

(2005) Controlled clinical trial of IV cyclophosphamide versus IV methylprednisolone in severe neurological manifestations in systemic lupus erythematosus. *Annals of the Rheumatic Diseases.* **64**(4): 620–5.

- Mawrin C, Brunn A, Rocken C and Schroder JM (2003) Peripheral neuropathy in systemic lupus erythematosus: pathomorphological features and distribution pattern of matrix metalloproteinases. *Acta Neuropathologica.* **105**(4): 365–72.

30 **False.**
Acute intermittent porphyria is the main form of porphyria in the UK. It is inherited in an autosomal dominant pattern and is secondary to reduced porphobilingen deaminase activity. Porphyria variegata is secondary to reduced protoporphyrinogen oxidase activity.

Reference:

- Burgovne K, Swartz R and Ananth J (1995) Porphyria: reexamination of psychiatric implications. *Psychotherapy and Psychosomatics.* **64**(3–4): 121–30.

---

31 The Continuous Performance Test (CPT) involves the presentation of target stimuli among random stimuli on a computer screen.

32 Personal construct theory emphasises man as a historian.

33 The Bedford College method of assessing life events allows both idiographic and nomothetic information to be combined.

34 Sleep disorders may be associated with HLA DR2.

35 The Bedford College method of assessing life events rates life events on a severity scale of 1 to 100.

---

31 **True.**
In the Continuous Performance Test a computer screen is used. The subject has to respond to predesignated stimuli on the screen that are presented transiently among rapidly changing random stimuli.

32 **False.**
George Kelly's personal construct theory supposes that man is a scientist who hypothesises about the world and tests out those hypotheses. Based on these experiments, man develops personal constructs which are bipoles, e.g. good self vs. bad self, trust vs. not-trust. Certain of these constructs are more important than others and are termed core constructs.

Reference:

- Kelly GA (1955) *The Psychology of Personal Constructs: Vols 1 and 2.* Norton, New York.

33 True.
The Bedford College method of assessing life events takes into account the social context of that event in measuring the impact on the individual, unlike many life-event scales and schedules. The event is assessed in terms of its *meaning* for the individual rather than how the individual reports that they felt at the time.

Reference:

● 　Brown GW and Harris T (1978) *Social Origins of Depression*. Tavistock, London.

34 True.
Almost all cases of narcolepsy have the HLA type DR2 (cf. 25% of the general population).

35 False.

---

36 High interdiagnoser reliability is a feature of a good diagnostic taxonomy.

37 The central tendency is another term for the standard deviation.

38 A *t*-test measures statistical significance of the distance between the means of two sets of scores.

39 A nominal measure has categories that are ranked, but not in terms of equal size.

40 The probability that a given result could be caused by sampling error is called the Z-score.

---

36 True.
For a good diagnostic taxonomy, reliability across time, between diagnosticians and between reporting sources (e.g. patient and informant) is important.

37 False.
The central tendency is the point in a distribution around which other scores tend to cluster.

38 True.

39 False.
An ordinal measure has categories that are ranked, but not in terms of equal size. A nominal measure has distinct categories that cannot be ranked.

40 **False.**
The probability that a given result could be caused by sampling error is called the statistical significance. The Z-score is a score minus the mean divided by the standard deviation.

---

41 The correlation measures the strength of association between two interval variables.

42 The Parental Bonding Instrument measures dependency.

43 Organic amnesia prevents learning through simple classical conditioning.

44 Lesions of the midline diencephalon can cause organic amnesia.

45 Prader-Willi syndrome is associated with an abnormal chromosome 11.

---

41 **True.**

42 **False.**
The Parental Bonding Instrument is a 25-item questionnaire given to patients who rate statements about their mother and father. It measures care and control, not dependency. 'Neurotic depressives' tend to give lower care scores and higher control scores to their parents.

Reference:

- Parker G, Tupling H and Brown LB (1979) A parental bonding instrument. *Br J Med Psychol.* **52**: 1–10.

43 **False.**
Simple classical conditioning can occur in cases of organic amnesia.

44 **True.**

Amnesia can be caused by independent lesions of the medial temporal lobes, midline diencephalons, and cholinergic basal forebrain.

Reference:

- Mayes A (1991) Amnesia: lesion location and functional deficit. *Psychol Med.* **21**: 293–7.

45 **False.**
Prader-Willi syndrome (PWS) is a complex human genetic disease that arises from lack of expression of paternally inherited imprinted genes on chromosome

15q11-q13. It is a rare cause (1%) of cases of learning disability. Prader-Willi cases are characterised by hypotonia, hyperphagia, and hypogenitalism.

Reference:

● Goldstone AP (2004) Prader-Willi syndrome: advances in genetics, pathophysiology and treatment. *Trends in Endocrinology and Metabolism.* **15**(1): 12–20.

---

46 A type 2 error occurs where there is no true association, but the p-value is significant.

47 The association between schizophrenia and low social class may be an example of reverse causality.

48 Perception at the absolute threshold is the highest intensity of a stimulus that can be tolerated.

49 Dichotic listening can help investigate selective attention.

50 Significant genetic linkage is implied by a lod score of less than 3.

---

46 False.
A type 1 error occurs when the p-value is so small that the null hypothesis can be rejected, but the association being studied arises by chance. A type 2 error occurs when a real association is missed because the variation is too large for the sample size.

47 True.
The association between some factor and a disease may be because the factor causes the disease, or it may be because the disease causes the factor, or some other intermediary link. A confounder is some factor associated with both the disease and the 'exposure' that can lead to a spurious association. For instance, if depression is found to be associated with smoking: is the smoking having direct effects on the brain, or might it be some confounding variable, e.g. chronic bronchitis?

48 False.
The absolute threshold is the lowest intensity of a stimulus that can be detected.

49 True.
In dichotic listening, two different messages are presented simultaneously through headphones and the subject is asked to pay attention to only one of the messages. The 'unattended' message is still processed by the brain though and attention can switch if its contents are of more interest, e.g. if the subject's name is mentioned in the 'unattended' message.

Reference:

● Treisman AM (1969) Strategies and models of selective attention. *Psychol Rev.* **76**: 282–99.

50 **False.**
In genetic linkage studies, the log of the odds score (lod score) for various values of the recombination fraction indicates significant linkage if it is greater than 3.

---

51 The standard notation for gene location uses the term 'p' to indicate the long arm of the chromosome.

52 Validity is a measure of a rating scale's ability to produce consistent results.

53 A so-called coverant behaviour is a covert operant behaviour.

54 Skinner's psychological theories only describe observable non-verbal behaviours.

55 Average rating scales achieve inter-rater reliability scores of approximately 0.9.

---

51 **False.**
In the notation for gene location, the first item is the chromosome number, the second whether the gene is on the short or long arm and the third the segment number of the arm where the gene is. In terms of which arm the gene is on, 'p' denotes the short arm and 'q' denotes the long arm.

52 **False.**
Validity is an assessment of whether a test or scale measures what it is supposed to. If there is a high correlation between the test score and the quality it is supposed to measure, then the test is said to be valid. Reliability is concerned with whether the scale or test can achieve consistent results.

53 **True.**
Lloyd Homme introduced the concept of coverant behaviour, a contraction of covert and operant, to describe the mental events or behaviours that mimic observable operant behaviour, such as intrusive thoughts.

Reference:

● Homme LE (1965) Perspectives in psychology: xxiv. Control of coverants: the operants of the mind. *Psychol Rec.* **15**: 501.

54 **False.**

BF Skinner wrote an account of the acquisition of language and the development of thought in *Verbal Behaviour* (1957). Skinner has made numerous contributions to behavioural psychology, including operant conditioning, the Skinner box, and shaping where behaviour is shaped by controlling the responses the environment makes to particular behaviours.

55 **False.**

Average rating scales achieve inter-rater reliability scores of approximately 0.6.

Reference:

● Hamilton M (1976) Comparative value of rating scales. *Br J Clin Pharmacol.* **Suppl.**: 58–60.

---

56 A behavioural response is much harder to extinguish if it was acquired during continuous rather than partial reinforcement.

57 Piaget was associated with developing the concept of object constancy.

58 The two-factor theory of intelligence was originated by Eysenck.

59 Ecstasy raises blood prolactin levels.

60 The incidence rate of a disorder is the number of completed episodes of illness in a year.

---

56 **False.**

Partial reinforcement occurs where a response is reinforced only some of the time. This makes it less likely to be extinguished when reinforcement eventually stops than if continuous reinforcement had been previously used.

Reference:

● Humphrey LG (1939) The effect of random alternation of re-inforcement on the acquisition and extinction of conditioned eyelid reactions. *J Exp Psychol.* **25**: 141–58.

57 **True.**

Piaget called his programme to study the development of children's intelligence 'genetic epistemology'. He described four stages of development of children's thought: sensori-motor, preoperational, concrete operations, and formal operational thought. Object constancy describes the ability to recognise the continued existence of an object even when it is out of the immediate arena of awareness.

58 **False.**
It was Spearman (1863–1945), an English psychologist, who coined the two-factor theory of intelligence, involving a general intelligence (g) and a task-specific intelligence (s).

59 **True.**

60 **False.**
The incidence rate is the number of episodes of ill health begun or people becoming ill in a specified time, over the number exposed to risk at the midpoint of the period.

---

61 The point prevalence rate is the number of illnesses at any time over the number of people exposed to risk in a period.

62 Parametric statistical methods include the chi-squared test.

63 Galactosaemia is inherited in an autosomal recessive fashion.

64 Sitting without support is accomplished by 80% of six-month-old infants.

65 The availability of tryptophan is rate limiting in the synthesis of serotonin.

---

61 **False.**
The point prevalence rate refers to a specific point in time not over a period of time.

62 **False.**
Parametric methods depend on assumptions made about distributions, e.g. Student's *t* distribution. Non-parametric methods are distribution-free, e.g the chi-squared test which is used for categorical data.

Reference:

● Norman GR and Streiner DL (2003) *PDQ Statistics* (3e). BC Decker, London.

63 **True.**
Galactosaemia involves a deficiency of galactose-1-phosphate uridyl transferase, resulting in retardation, hepatomegaly and cataracts. A galactose-free diet is effective if started early.

64 **False.**
Sitting without support is accomplished by 50% of children at six months.

65 **True.**

66 Most of the 5-HT released in the CNS originates from the cells of the Raphe nuclei of the brainstem and mid-brain.

67 Bromocriptine increases the release of DA (dopamine) from the presynaptic vesicles.

68 The spinothalamic pathway terminates in the nucleus gracilis and nucleus cuneatus.

69 Noradrenaline is formed by the hydroxylation of L-tryptophan.

70 Convergent validity is held to be established when measures that are predicted to be associated are found not to be related.

66 **True.**

67 **False.**
Bromocriptine is a dopamine agonist acting mainly at post-synaptic D2 receptors.

68 **False.**
The spinothalamic tract terminates in the ventro post lateral nucleus of the thalamus.

69 **False.**
Serotonin is formed by the hydroxylation of L-tryptophan to 5-hydroxy-tryptophan which is then decarboxylated to 5-hydroxytryptamine.

70 **False.**
Convergent validity occurs when measures that are predicted to be associated are found to be related (i.e. measure the same thing), as opposed to divergent validity where measures successfully discriminate between unrelated constructs.

Reference:

- American Psychological Association (1954) Technical recommendations for psychological tests and diagnostic techniques. *Psychol Bull.* **Suppl. 51**(part 2): 1–38.

71 Neurofibrillary tangles are composed mainly of tau proteins.

72 Vasoactive intestinal peptide is also a cortical neuropeptide.

73 In adults delta waves on the EEG (electro-encephalogram) become more obvious with relaxation and drowsiness.

74 The hypothalamus has osmoreceptors to detect increased osmotic pressure in the carotid blood supply.

75 The hypothalamus controls the neurosecretory cells of the adeno-hypophysis via the neurohypophysial tract.

71 **True.**

References:

- Gomez-Ramos P and Moran MA (1998) Ultrastructural aspects of neuro-fibrillary tangle formation in aging and Alzheimer's disease. *Microscopy Research and Technique.* **43**(1): 49–58.
- Peskind ER (1996) Neurobiology of Alzheimer's disease. *Journal of Clinical Psychiatry.* **57** (suppl. 14): 5–8.

72 **True.**
Vasoactive intestinal peptide (VIP) has been shown to be neuroprotective and to play a role in learning and memory.

Reference:

- Pinhasov A, Mandel S, Torchinsky A, Giladi E, Pittel Z, Goldsweig AM, Servoss SJ, Brenneman DE and Gozes I (2003) Activity-dependent neuroprotective protein: a novel gene essential for brain formation. *Brain Research. Developmental Brain Research.* **144**(1): 83–90.

73 **True.**
Delta waves are diffusely distributed and normally seen only in sleeping adults and in children.

74 **True.**
Osmoreceptors in the perinuclear areas stimulate cells of the supraoptic and periventricular nuclei to stop the release of antidiuretic hormone.

75 **False.**
The neurohypophysial tract has neural connections with the posterior pituitary rather than the adenohypophysis (anterior pituitary).

76 The hypothalamus has output fibres in the principal mamillar fasciculus.

77 The term 'theory of mind' was first introduced to help understand the cognitive and language abilities of chimpanzees.

78 Children are capable of sustaining pretend play with peers at around three years of age.

79 Macrosystems, exosystems, microsystems and chronosystems are associated with the concept of ecological development.

80 Research data suggest that SSRIs are highly effective in the treatment of depression in childhood and adolescence.

76 **True.**

77 **True.**

Reference:

● Premack D and Woodruff G (1978) Does the chimpanzee have a theory of mind? *Behavioural and Brain Sciences.* **1**: 515–26.

78 **True.**

Reference:

● Garvey C (1977) *Play.* Harvard, Cambridge.

79 **True.**
Bronfenbrenner is closely associated with the increased recognition of the influence of environmental context on children's development.

Reference:

● Bronfenbrenner U (1981) *The Ecology of Human Development.* Harvard University Press, Cambridge.

80 **False.**
Results of studies are equivocal. The evidence base is strongest for fluoxetine and published studies tend to report more favourable outcomes than unpublished studies.

Reference:

● Whittington CJ *et al.* (2004) SSRIs in childhood depression. *The Lancet.* **363**(9418): 1341–5.

81 Autism is a *moderately* heritable condition.

82 The prevalence of depression in prepubertal children is approximately 6%.

83 Initial studies suggesting that the neuregulin-1 gene is implicated in schizophrenia have not been replicated.

84 The Alzheimer Disease Assessment Scale – cognitive section (ADAS-COG) is widely used to evaluate change in cognitive function in drug trials for Alzheimer's disease.

85 Late-onset schizophrenia is accompanied by a deterioration of cognitive performance similar to that seen in neurodegenerative dementia.

81 **False.**
Autism is highly heritable, with estimates of heritability around 90%.

Reference:

- Bespalova IN and Buxbaum JD (2003) Disease susceptibility genes for autism. *Ann Med.* 35(4): 274–81.

82 **False.**
The prevalence of depression is approximately 0.5–2.5% in prepubertal children, rising to 2–8% during adolescence.

Reference:

- Lask B, Taylor S and Nunn K (2003) *Practical Child Psychiatry. The clinician's guide.* BMJ Publishing Group, London.

83 **False.**
Several studies have provided evidence that variation at the neuregulin 1 (NRG1) gene on chromosome 8p12 influences susceptibility to schizophrenia. Further studies have suggested that neuregulin 1 plays a role in influencing susceptibility to bipolar disorder and schizophrenia and that it may exert a specific effect in the subset of functional psychosis that has manic and mood-incongruent psychotic features.

Reference:

- Green EK, Raybould R, Macgregor S, Gordon-Smith K, Heron J, Hyde S, Grozeva D, Hamshere M, Williams N, Owen MJ, O'Donovan MC, Jones L, Jones I, Kirov G and Craddock N (2005) Operation of the schizophrenia susceptibility gene, neuregulin 1, across traditional diagnostic boundaries to increase risk for bipolar disorder. *Archives of General Psychiatry.* 62(6): 642–8.

84 True.

Reference:

● Rosen W, Mohs R and Davis KL (1984) A new rating scale for Alzheimer's disease. *American Journal of Psychiatry.* **141**: 135–64.

85 False.
Neuropsychological findings in late-onset schizophrenia include impaired performance on measures of executive function, learning, motor skills and verbal ability which are quantitatively and qualitatively different from those seen in dementia.

Reference:

● Howard R *et al.* (2000) Late onset and very late onset schizophrenia-like psychosis: an international consensus. *American Journal of Psychiatry.* **157**: 172–8.

---

86 The type of memory that shows the greatest decrement with normal ageing is implicit memory.

87 There is supplementary normative data for the Wechsler Adult Intelligence Scale for individuals up to 96 years of age.

88 Subcortical dementia is characterised by difficulties with the encoding and consolidation of new information.

89 Aphasia, agnosia and apraxia are commonly seen in Huntington's disease.

90 Hypomania is more common after left cerebral hemisphere stroke than right.

---

86 False.
The largest decrements are observed in recent, episodic memory. Implicit memory is reasonably stable with age.

Reference:

● Prull MW, Gabrieli JDE and Bunge SA (2000) Age related changes in memory: a neuroscience perspective. In: FM Craik and TA Salthouse (eds) *Handbook of Ageing and Cognition* (2e). Erlbaum, Mahwah, NJ.

87 True.

Reference:

- Koltain DC and Welsh-Bonner KA (2000) Geriatric neuropsychological assessment. In: RD Vanderploeg (ed.) *Clinician's Guide to Neuropsychological Assessment* (2e). Lawrence Erlbaum Associates, Mahweh, NJ.

88 **False.**
Cortical dementia, like Alzheimer's disease, is characterised by problems with encoding and consolidation of new information, while subcortical disorders, including depression, are conceptualised as resulting in retrieval deficits despite adequate storage of information.

Reference:

- Cummings J and Benson D (1992) *Dementia: a clinical approach*. Butterworth-Heinemann, Stoneham, MA.

89 **False.**
These are uncommon. Cognitive impairment comprises loss of memory, calculation, verbal fluency, visuospatial and executive functioning.

Reference:

- Naarding P *et al.* (2001) Huntington's disease: a review of the literature on prevalence and treatment of neuropsychiatric phenomena. *European Psychiatry.* **16**: 439–45.

90 **False.**
A hypomanic picture is more frequent after right hemispheric stroke as compared to left.

Reference:

- Starkstein S *et al.* (1988) Mechanisms of mania after brain injury. *Journal of Nervous and Mental Disease.* **176**: 87–100.

---

91 The most consistent and widely described structural change in patients with a clinical diagnosis of Alzheimer's disease is atrophy of medial temporal lobe structures.

92 Late-onset schizophrenia occurs equally in men and women.

93 Parietal lobe tumours are typically associated with gustatory and olfactory hallucinations.

94 There is no difference in the prevalence of vascular dementia between black Afro-Caribbean and white British older adults.

95 Late-onset mania has a lower incidence of family history of affective disorder than early-onset mania.

91 True.

Reference:

- O'Brien J and Barber B (2000) Neuroimaging in depression and dementia. *Advances in Psychiatric Treatment.* **6**: 109–19.

92 False.
There is marked preponderance for women. Studies have shown the F:M ratio to range from 9:1 to 4:1. The later the age of onset, the greater the proportion of women affected.

Reference:

- Anderson N and Jacques A (2004) *Companion to Psychiatric Studies* (7e). Churchill Livingstone, Edinburgh, Chapter 26.

93 False.
Parietal lobe tumours are associated with localised tactile and kinaesthetic hallucinations. Occipital lobe tumours are associated with visual hallucinations. Temporal lobe tumours are associated with gustatory, olfactory, visual and auditory hallucinations. These distinctions are however not absolute.

Reference:

- Lishman WA (1998) *Organic Psychiatry* (3e). Blackwell, London, Chapter 6, p.219.

94 False.
Black older people are significantly more likely to have vascular dementia than white British older people and there is an increased frequency of stroke, diabetes and hypertension in the black population. The increased risk of vascular dementia is around 12 times.

Reference:

- Livingston G and Sembhi S (2003) Mental health of the ageing immigrant population. *Advances in Psychiatric Treatment.* **9**: 31–7.

95 True.
Late-onset mania is associated with cerebral pathology, often vascular with right hemispheric lesions predominating. Such organic factors may explain why patients with late-onset mania have lower incidence of family history of affective disorder.

Reference:

- Braun CM *et al.* (1999) Mania, pseudomania, depression and pseudodepression resulting from focal unilateral cortical lesions. *Neuropsychiatry, Neuropsychology and Behavioural Neurology.* **12**: 35–51.

96 The Wechsler Adult Intelligence Scale (WAIS) includes a test of vocabulary.
97 Cognitive-analytic therapy was developed by Aaron Beck.
98 Carbamazepine and sodium valproate can be given once daily because they are slowly metabolised.
99 In child psychotherapy the mother–infant relationship is the paradigm for the analytic process, according to Winnicott.
100 Psychiatric symptoms are often the first presenting feature of anteriorly placed frontal lobe tumours.

96 **True.**
The Wechsler Adult Intelligence Scale (WAIS) has 11 sub-tests divided between verbal and performance tests. Verbal sub-tests include information, comprehension, arithmetic, similarities, digit span, and vocabulary. Performance sub-tests include digit symbol, picture completion, block design, picture arrangement, and object assembly. The WAIS gives an intelligence quotient, and has a role in identifying brain damage by showing discrepancies between verbal and performance IQs.

Reference:

- Wechsler D (1958) *The Measurement and Appraisal of Adult Intelligence* (4e). Williams and Wilkins, Baltimore.

97 **False.**
Cognitive behavioural therapy was derived from Beck's work. Cognitive analytic therapy was developed by Anthony Ryle.

References:

- Beck AT (1976) *Cognitive Therapy and the Emotional Disorders*. International Universities Press, New York.
- Ryle A (1991) *Cognitive-Analytic Therapy: active participation in change*. John Wiley, Chichester.

98 **False.**
In the management of epilepsy carbamazepine and sodium valproate need to be given several times daily as they are rapidly metabolised.

99 **True.**
Winnicott saw interpretation in analytic treatment as a sophisticated extension of infant care, and therefore an echo of the mother–infant relationship.

References:

- Winnicott D (1986) *Holding and Interpretation: fragment of an analysis*. Hogarth Press, London.

- Winnicott D (1971) *Therapeutic Consultation in Child Psychiatry*. Hogarth Press, London.

100 **True.**
Psychiatric symptoms are the first to appear in anteriorly placed frontal lobe tumours in over a third of cases.

Reference:

- Ron MA (1989) Psychiatric manifestations of frontal lobe tumours. *Br J Psychiatry*. **155**: 735–8.

Extended Matching Item

Q1 Assessment in child psychiatry:

A ADOS
B Stroop test
C ADI
D 3Di
E PACS
F K-SADS
G CARS
H DISCO
J PICA

An eight-year-old boy is referred by his GP. His parents complain that he has abnormal speech and mixes up his words. He has no friends, can't follow simple instructions and often refuses to do what is asked. His behaviour is difficult and at school he cannot sit still.

1 You are concerned he may have an autistic spectrum disorder. Which assessment(s) could you use to directly examine the child?
2 You are concerned he may have an autistic spectrum disorder. Which assessment(s) could you use to interview the parents?
3 Which assessment(s) could you use with the parents to look at symptoms of ADHD?

A1

1 Answer A.
   ADOS – Autism Diagnostic Observational Schedule.

2 Answer C, D and H.
   ADI – Autism Diagnostic Interview.
   3Di – Developmental, Dimensional and Diagnostic interview.
   DISCO – Diagnostic Interview for Social and Communication disorder
   (Lorna Wing).

3 Answer E.
   PACS – Parent Account of Childhood Symptoms (Eric Taylor).

MRCPsych Part II: Clinical Topics Written Paper

Individual Statements

---

1 Male adolescents with moderate/severe reading disorders are at increased risk of developing schizophrenia.

2 Increasing age is a risk factor for developing hyponatraemia while taking selective serotonin reuptake inhibitor (SSRI) antidepressants.

3 Rivastigmine is a drug treatment for mild and moderate Alzheimer's disease that acts as an inhibitor of the enzyme acetylcholinesterase and has a modulatory effect on nicotinic acetylcholine receptors.

4 People over 80 years of age who take antidepressants with high inhibition of serotonin reuptake are at increased risk of gastrointestinal haemorrhage because these drugs inhibit the uptake of serotonin by platelets.

5 Cognitive behavioural therapy is ineffective in children of primary school age.

---

1 True.
In general, and particularly with males, people with schizophrenia show significant premorbid deficits on all intellectual and behavioural measures and on measures of reading and reading comprehension.

References:

● Vourdas A, Pipe R, Corrigall R and Frangou S (2003) Increased developmental deviance and premorbid dysfunction in early onset schizophrenia. *Schizophrenia Research.* **62**(1–2): 13–22.

- Reichenberg A *et al.* (2002) A population-based cohort study of premorbid intellectual, language, and behavioral functioning in patients with schizophrenia, schizoaffective disorder, and nonpsychotic bipolar disorder. *American Journal of Psychiatry.* **159**(12): 2027–35.

2   **True.**

Reference:

- Kirby D and Ames D (2001) Hyponatraemia and selective serotonin reuptake inhibitors in elderly patients. *International Journal of Geriatric Psychiatry.* **16**: 484–93.

3   **False.**
Galantamine is the only acetylcholinesterase inhibitor known to have a modulatory effect on nicotinic receptors though the clinical significance of this effect is uncertain.

Reference:

- *International Psychogeriatrics* (2002) **14** (Supplement 1) gives a thorough review of cholinesterase inhibitors.

4   **True.**
Serotonin potentiates platelet aggregation and serotonin reuptake inhibitors decrease the serotonin uptake by platelets from the blood.

Reference:

- van Walraven C, Mamdani MM, Wells PS and Williams JI (2001) Inhibition of serotonin reuptake by antidepressants and upper gastrointestinal bleeding in elderly patients: retrospective cohort study. *BMJ.* **323**: 655–8.

5   **False.**
For CBT to be effective in children, they must be cognitively able to use the strategies employed in therapy. This is unlikely to occur before the age of seven, but has occurred by the age of 10 in most children.

Reference:

- Lask B, Taylor S and Nunn K (2003) *Practical Child Psychiatry. The clinician's guide.* BMJ Publishing Group, London.

6 Methylphenidate has been used in the treatment of ADHD for over 40 years.

7 Children with conduct disorder are more likely to be living in lone-parent families when compared with those without a mental disorder.

8 Electrocardiograms should be regularly checked in children taking atomoxetine.

9 A good outcome for ECT treatment of depression can be predicted if there is evidence of psychomotor retardation and psychosis.

10 According to research evidence ECT for depression with continuation antidepressants has a superior long-term outcome to ECT for depression without continuation antidepressants.

6 **True.**
Methylphenidate has been used in treating ADHD since 1957.

Reference:

- Greenhill L (1995) *Child Adolesc Psychiatric Clin N Am.* 4(1): 123–68.

7 **True.**
Forty-two per cent of children with conduct disorders live in lone-parent families compared with 21% of children without mental disorder.

Reference:

- Meltzer H and Gatward R (1999) *Mental Health of Children and Adolescents in Britain.* National Statistics Office, London.

8 **False.**
There has been no evidence of atomoxetine affecting the Q-Tc interval, or of other ECG (electrocardiogram) changes. Atomoxetine is associated with mild increases in pulse rate and blood pressure during treatment.

Reference:

- Kratochvil C *et al.* (2003) Atomoxetine: a selective noradrenaline reuptake inhibitor for the treatment of attention-deficit/hyperactivity disorder. *Expert Opin Pharmacother.* 4(7): 1165–74.

9 **True.**

Reference:

- Petrides G, Fink M, Husain MM *et al.* (2001) ECT remission rates in psychotic versus nonpsychotic depressed patients: a report from CORE. *Journal of ECT.* **17**(4): 244–53.

10 **True.**
Without active treatment, virtually all (>80%) remitted patients relapse within six months of stopping ECT.

Reference:

- Sackeim HA, Haskett RF, Mulsant BH *et al.* (2001) Continuation pharmacotherapy in the prevention of relapse following electroconvulsive therapy: a randomized controlled trial. *JAMA.* **285**(10): 1299–307.

---

11 There is no research evidence to support the long-term use of maintenance ECT.

12 Clozapine response can be predicted with over 70% success using a combination of polymorphisms in neuroreceptor-related genes.

13 There is an evidence base for the treatment of Tourette's syndrome with rTMS (repetitive transcranial magnetic stimulation).

14 Episodic anxiety has been linked to abnormal blood flow in the right hippocampal area.

15 Episodic anxiety usually remits completely within a year of diagnosis.

---

11 **False.**
Gagne *et al.* identified 29 patients who received continuation ECT plus long-term antidepressant treatment after a positive response to acute treatment with ECT for a depressive episode (forming a continuation ECT group). They used a retrospective case-controlled approach to obtain a matching group of 29 patients who just received long-term antidepressants after responding positively to acute ECT. The cumulative probability of surviving without relapse or recurrence at two years was 93% for continuation ECT patients and 52% for antidepressant-alone patients.

Reference:

- Gagne GG Jr, Furman MJ, Carpenter LL and Price LH (2000) Efficacy of continuation ECT and antidepressant drugs compared to long-term antidepressants alone in depressed patients. *American Journal of Psychiatry.* **157**(12): 1960–5.

12 **True.**
Association studies in multiple candidate genes found a combination of polymorphisms in neurotransmitter receptor-related genes giving 76.7% success in the prediction of clozapine response (p=0.0001) and a sensitivity of 95% (+/– 0.04) for satisfactory response in schizophrenia.

Reference:

- Arranz MJ, Munro J, Birkett J *et al.* (2000) Pharmacogenetic prediction of clozapine response. *The Lancet.* 355(9215): 1615–16.

13 **False.**

Reference:

- Stern JS, Burza S and Robertson MM (2005) Gilles de la Tourette's syndrome and its impact in the UK. *Postgraduate Medical Journal.* 81(951): 12–19.

14 **True.**
Positron emission tomography studies have shown an increase in blood flow in the right parahippocampal area.

Reference:

- Reiman EM *et al.* (1986) The application of positron emission tomography to the study of panic disorder. *Am J Psychiatr.* 143: 469.

15 **False.**
In a study of neurotic illness in general practice, only 24% of neurotic illness had improved over one year (25% had a variable course and 25% a chronic course). It is therefore untrue to suggest that episodic anxiety *usually completely* remits within one year.

Reference:

- Mann AH, Jenkins R and Belsey E (1981) The 12-month outcome of patients with neurotic illness in general practice. *Psychol Med.* 11: 535–50.

---

16 Huntington's disease usually presents in the third decade of life.

17 Deep brain stimulation (DBS) has been used in treatment-resistant depression and intractable obsessive-compulsive disorder (OCD).

18 CBT for depression has residual effects which prevent relapse, but this effect fades after just six months.

19 Naltrexone (NTX) treatment can lower the risk of treatment withdrawal in most alcohol-dependent patients.

20 The fragile-X syndrome may present with language delay.

16 **False.**
Huntington's disease was first described in 1872 and has been localised to chromosome 4. It has complete penetrance in hereditary terms. Pre-symptomatic testing has a small margin of error (about 2%). It usually presents in the fifth decade of life. The duration of the illness is 13 to 16 years.

Reference:

● Lishman WA (1998) *Organic Psychiatry* (3e). Blackwell, London.

17 **True.**
Deep brain stimulation (DBS) was originally investigated for use in Parkinson's disease. It has been found to be useful in some small studies with cases of treatment-resistant depression and intractable obsessive-compulsive disorder. DBS is used in depression to modulate supposed overactivity of the subgenual cingulate region (Brodmann area 25). The treatment is currently experimental.

Reference:

● Mayberg HS, Lozano AM, Voon V, McNeely HE, Seminowicz D, Hamani C, Schwalb JM and Kennedy SH (2005) Deep brain stimulation for treatment-resistant depression. *Neuron.* **45**(5): 651–60.

18 **False.**
The effect of CBT in reduction of relapse and recurrence persists for several years. Paykel *et al.* (2005) conducted a randomised controlled trial of CBT plus medication and clinical management versus medication and clinical management alone, followed six years after randomisation. Effects in prevention of relapse and recurrence were found to persist, with weakening, and were not fully lost until $3\frac{1}{2}$ years after the end of therapy.

Reference:

● Paykel ES, Scott J, Cornwall PL, Abbott R, Crane C, Pope M and Johnson AL (2005) Duration of relapse prevention after cognitive therapy in residual depression: follow-up of controlled trial. *Psychological Medicine.* **35**(1): 59–68.

19 **False.**
NTX treatment can lower the risk of treatment withdrawal in 28% of alcohol-dependent patients.

Reference:

● Srisurapanont M and Jarusuraisin N (2005) Opioid antagonists for alcohol dependence. [Update of *Cochrane Database Syst Rev* (2002). **2**: CD001867; PMID: 12076425.] *Cochrane Database of Systematic Reviews.* **1**: CD001867.

20 **True.**

21 Tourette's syndrome is usually caused by childhood streptococcal infections.

22 Nocturnal sleep is mainly composed of REM (rapid eye movement) sleep.

23 Brain lesions in the posterior right hemisphere are associated with prosopagnosia.

24 Brain lesions only cause constructional apraxia when they are in the right parietal lobe.

25 Twenty per cent of males inheriting a fragile-X chromosome are asymptomatic.

21 **False.**
There is some evidence linking Tourette's with streptococcal infections, but there also appears to be a strong genetic aetiology and so the causation appears to be heterogenous.

References:

- Hoekstra PJ, Anderson GM, Limburg PC, Korf J, Kallenberg CG and Minderaa RB (2004) Neurobiology and neuroimmunology of Tourette's syndrome: an update. *Cellular and Molecular Life Sciences.* **61**(7–8): 886–98.
- Kerbeshian J, Burd L and Pettit R (1990) A possible post-streptococcal movement disorder with chorea and tics. *Developmental Medicine and Child Neurology.* **32**(7): 642–4.

22 **False.**
Eighty per cent of night-time sleep is filled by orthodox or non-REM sleep.

23 **True.**
Prosopagnosia implies an impairment in facial recognition

Reference:

- McCarthy RA and Warrington EK (1990) *Cognitive Neuropsychology.* Academic Press Inc, California.

24 **False.**
Constructional apraxias can occur in left and right hemispheric lesions, but there is a *qualitative* difference between right and left hemispheric constructional apraxias. For instance, on the drawing test of copying a house picture, right hemisphere lesions lead to a so-called 'exploded' diagram, whereas left hemisphere lesions produce 'oversimplified' diagrams.

25 **True.**

26 In Huntington's disease the age of onset is much earlier if it is inherited from the mother.

27 Ecstasy induces a hypertensive crisis if taken with MAOIs (monoamine oxidase inhibitors).

28 Tuberous sclerosis is inherited in an autosomal recessive fashion.

29 There is good evidence that Reminiscence Therapy improves the behavioural symptoms of dementia.

30 Interpersonal therapy has been shown to be effective for relapse prevention of depression in older people.

26 **False.**

Huntington's disease has been repeatedly found to have an earlier age of onset if inherited from the male, and has been cited as an example of genomic imprinting. In genomic imprinting the severity of expression of a genetic disease is affected by whether the particular chromosomes are derived from maternal or paternal sources. The problem is related to expanded repeats of gene sequences in paternal transmission. The effect is also cited in neurofibromatosis, myotonic dystrophy, fragile-X disease, and cerebellar ataxia.

References:

- Bird ED, Caro AJ and Pilling JB (1974) A sex-related factor in the inheritance of Huntington's chorea. *Ann Hum Genet.* **37**: 255–60.
- Chatkupt S, Antonowicz M and Johnson WG (1995) Parents do matter: genomic imprinting and parental sex effects in neurological disorders. *Journal of the Neurological Sciences.* **130**(1): 1–10.

27 **True.**

28 **False.**

Tuberous sclerosis is an autosomal dominant condition.

29 **False.**

There is good evidence that Reality Orientation improves the cognitive and behavioural symptoms of dementia but not Reminiscence Therapy. For a good account of the management of the behavioural and psychological symptoms of dementia, *see* Ballard *et al.* (2001).

References:

- Ballard CG, O'Brien J, James I and Swann A (2001) *Dementia: management of behavioural and psychological symptoms.* Oxford University Press, Oxford.

- Spector A, Orrell M, Davies S *et al.* (2002) Reality Orientation for dementia. *Cochrane Library.* Issue 3. Update Software, Oxford.
- Spector A, Orrell M, Davies S *et al.* (2002) Reminiscence Therapy for dementia. *Cochrane Library.* Issue 3. Update Software, Oxford.

30 **True.**
For a thorough review of psychotherapies for older people, *see* Hepple *et al.* (2002).

References:

- Hepple JN, Pearce J and Wilkinson PW (eds) (2002) *Psychological Therapies with Older People; developing treatments for effective practice.* Brunner-Routledge, Hove.
- Reynolds III C *et al.* (1999) Nortryptiline and interpersonal psychotherapy as maintenance therapies for recurrent major depression: a randomised controlled trial in patients older than 59 years. *JAMA.* **281**: 39–45.

---

31 Hyperorality is a core feature of Fronto Temporal Dementia (FTD).

32 In Charles Bonnet syndrome patients experience visual hallucinations linked to visual impairment with complete loss of insight.

33 Left temporal dysfunction is often present in Capgras syndrome.

34 Thirty per cent of patients with Parkinson's disease develop hallucinations within the first five years of diagnosis.

35 Most of the variance in seizure threshold for ECT can be predicted by factors such as age or baldness.

---

31 **False.**
The core features of FTD comprise insidious onset and gradual progression, early decline in social and interpersonal conduct, emotional blunting and early loss of insight. The supportive features include mental rigidity, distractibility, hyperorality, perseveration and stereotypy of talk and behaviour, progressive reduction of speech output, echolalia with preserved praxis, spatial orientation and receptive speech. Physical signs include early incontinence, primitive reflexes, late akinesia, rigidity and tremor, low and labile blood pressure.

References:

- Anderson N and Jacques A (2004) *Companion to Psychiatric Studies* (7e). Churchill Livingstone, Edinburgh, Chapter 26, p.634.
- Snowden JS, Neary D and Mann DMA (2002) Fronto temporal dementia. *British Journal of Psychiatry.* **180**: 140–3.

32 **False.**
Partial or complete insight is retained in this syndrome.

Reference:

- Berrios GE and Brook P (1984) Visual hallucination and sensory delusion in the elderly. *British Journal of Psychiatry.* **144**: 652–64.

33 **False.**
In this syndrome the patient believes that a relative or friend has been replaced by an impostor who resembles the original exactly. It is associated with brain damage in almost two-thirds of cases and right fronto-temporal dysfunction appeared to be involved.

Reference:

- Malloy P, Cimino C and Westlake R (1992) Differential diagnoses of primary and secondary Capgras syndrome. *Neuropsychiatry, Neuropsychology and Behavioural Neurology.* **5**(15): 83–96.

34 **True.**

Reference:

- Fenelon G, Mahieux F, Huon R and Ziegler M (2000) Hallucinations in Parkinson's disease: prevalence, phenomenology and risk factors. *Brain.* **123**: 733–45.

35 **False.**
Only about 28% of variance can be predicted by factors such as age, sex and baldness.

---

36 There is substantial evidence from randomised controlled trials (RCTs) for the efficacy of transcranial magnetic stimulation in treating depressive disorder.

37 Suicide is associated with motor restlessness in schizophrenia.

38 The fragile-X syndrome is associated with repetitions of the base sequence CGG at the fragile site.

39 Loneliness is a risk factor for depression in later life.

40 Damage to the subcortical areas can result in reduplicative paramnesia.

---

36 **False.**
A recent meta-analysis suggested that rapid-rate rTMS is no different from sham treatment in major depression. A Cochrane analysis does not support

efficacy in treating depression. In addition there are currently insufficient data from randomised controlled trials to draw any conclusions about the efficacy of transcranial magnetic stimulation in the treatment of obsessive-compulsive disorder.

References:

- Couturier JL (2005) Efficacy of rapid-rate repetitive transcranial magnetic stimulation in the treatment of depression: a systematic review and meta-analysis. *Journal of Psychiatry and Neuroscience.* **30**(2): 83–90.
- Martin JL, Barbanoj MJ, Perez V and Sacristan M (2003) Transcranial magnetic stimulation for the treatment of obsessive-compulsive disorder. *Cochrane Database of Systematic Reviews.* **3**: CD003387.
- Martin JL, Barbanoj MJ, Schlaepfer TE, Clos S, Perez V, Kulisevsky J and Gironell A (2002) Transcranial magnetic stimulation for treating depression. *Cochrane Database of Systematic Reviews.* **2**: CD003493.

37 **True.**
Agitation or motor restlessness is associated with an increased risk of suicide (odds ratio 2.61).

Reference:

- Hawton, K, Sutton L, Haw, C, Sinclair, J and Deeks, JJ (2005) Schizophrenia and suicide: a systematic review of risk factors. *Br J Psychiatry.* **187**: 9–20.

38 **True.**
The fragile-X syndrome represents 20–30% of all cases of mental retardation. The syndrome, first recognised by Martin Bell, is associated with long faces, large ears, macro-orchidism and mild-to-moderate mental retardation. One-third of heterozygote females are intellectually impaired. Heterozygote females also are more prone to schizophrenia and affective disorder. Recent work has focused on the integral role of multiple CGG nucleotide arrays at the fragile site at the distal end of the X chromosome's long arm. These multiple arrays of CGG can be detected by direct DNA tests prenatally.

39 **True.**
Smoking, loneliness, lack of satisfaction with life and female sex all appeared to act as independent vulnerability factors for the genesis of depression three years later in the Liverpool Continuing Health in the Community Study. Bereavement of a close figure in the previous six months appeared to act as a trigger factor for cases of depression in the community (Green *et al.*, 1992).

Reference:

- Green BH, Copeland JRM, Dewey ME *et al.* (1992) Risk factors for depression in elderly people: a prospective study. *Acta Psychiatr Scand.* **86**: 213–17.

40 **False.**

Reduplicative paramnesia, which might involve someone maintaining that they are simultaneously at home and in the hospital, is attributable to a lesion of the parietal lobe.

---

41 There is no difference in severity of white matter lesions when comparing brains of late-onset older depressed patients and early-onset depressed older adults.

42 Severe dementia is a rare feature of progressive supranuclear palsy (PSP).

43 First-rank symptoms are seen in only 30% of cases of late-onset schizophrenia.

44 Bilateral ECT is more effective than unilateral ECT, and high-dose ECT is more effective than low-dose.

45 Negative reinforcement is an example of an operant technique.

---

41 **False.**

MRI visualised white matter lesions are greater in older depressed patients than controlled subjects. They are also greater in late-onset as compared to early-onset depression seen in older adults.

References:

- Baldwin RC (2005) Is vascular depression a distinct sub-type of depressive disorder? A review of causal evidence. *International Journal of Geriatric Psychiatry.* **20**: 1–11.
- Tupler LA *et al.* (2002) Anatomic location and laterality of MRI signal hyper intensities in late-life depression. *J Psychosomatic Res.* **53**: 665–76.

42 **True.**

The clinical features of PSP include gait instability, frequent falls, rigidity, erect posture with retrocollis, infrequent blinking and later dysarthria and dysphagia. Psychiatric features include bradyphrenia (mental slowing), irritability, social withdrawal and fatigability. Depression and emotional incontinence is also seen. Frontal lobe dysfunction may be striking but severe dementia is rare.

Reference:

- Rajput A and Rajput AH (2001) Progressive supranuclear palsy: clinical features, pathophysiology and management. *Drugs and Aging.* **18**: 913–25.

43 **True.**
Bleuler first described the term 'late-onset schizophrenia' in 1943 as occurring in individuals over the age of 40 without organic brain disease and having symptoms indistinguishable from schizophrenia at an earlier age.

44 **True.**
In a meta-analysis of studies bilateral ECT was deemed more effective than unipolar ECT (22 trials, 1408 participants, SES –0.32, 95% CI –0.46 to –0.19) and high-dose ECT more effective than low-dose.

Reference:

- UK ECT Review Group (2003) Efficacy and safety of electroconvulsive therapy in depressive disorders: a systematic review and meta-analysis. *The Lancet.* **361**(9360): 799–808.

45 **True.**
Operant conditioning is a type of learning in which behaviours are increased or decreased as a function of the events that follow them, i.e. reinforce them. Operant techniques also include extinction and punishing.

---

46 Bullies are typically bigger and stronger than their targets.

47 Lazarus's cognitive appraisal theory (1966) states that emotion is the cognitive appraisal of an emotional experience.

48 Homeostasis is a feature of systemic family therapy.

49 In ICD-10 specific speech articulation disorder is classed as a developmental disorder of scholastic skills.

50 According to Bentovim (1986) successful families should include mutual dependency and investment.

---

46 **True.**

Reference:

- Olweus D (1993) *Bullying At School.* Blackwell, Cambridge, MA.

47 **True.**
There are three stages to this theory: primary appraisal (which identifies emotional experience), secondary appraisal of behavioural responses and finally reappraisal.

References:

- Lau R and Morse CA (2001) Parents' coping in the neonatal intensive care unit: a theoretical framework. *Journal of Psychosomatic Obstetrics and Gynecology.* 22(1): 41–7.
- Thornton PI (1992) The relation of coping, appraisal, and burnout in mental health workers. *Journal of Psychology.* 126(3): 261–71.

48 True.

Systems theory was described by von Bertalaffny in 1973. Homeostasis is the mechanism where a system (family) in steady state will compensate for any change, or resist attempts to impose or create change.

Reference:

- von Bertalaffny L (1973) *General Systems Theory. Foundations, development, applications.* George Braziller, New York.

49 False.

Specific speech articulation disorder is found in disorders of speech and language.

50 False.

Successful families, according to Bentovim, provide a model for socialisation, models in the parents for sexual identity, and boundaries demarcating parents and children.

Reference:

- Bentovim A (1986) Family therapy. In: S Bloch S (ed.) *Introduction to the Psychotherapies.* Oxford Medical Publications, Oxford.

---

51 Deliberate self-harm as defined by Morgan (1979) does not include self-poisoning.

52 Senile dementia of the Lewy body type involves substantial loss of cells in the substantia nigra.

53 Therapeutic factors in small group psychotherapy include vicarious learning.

54 Methods of reducing unwanted behaviour include cue exposure.

55 Phenylketonuria can only be treated by total exclusion of phenylalanine from the diet in childhood.

51 **False.**

Morgan's (1979) definition of deliberate self-harm included both enteral and parenteral causes, and therefore included self-poisoning.

Reference:

- Douglas J, Cooper J, Amos T, Webb R, Guthrie E and Appleby L (2004) 'Near-fatal' deliberate self-harm: characteristics, prevention and implications for the prevention of suicide. *Journal of Affective Disorders.* **79**(1–3): 263–8.

52 **True.**

Senile dementia of the Lewy body type involves up to 40% of cells being lost from the substantia nigra. In Parkinson's disease up to 70% of cells in the substantia nigra must be lost before symptoms manifest. Even so, this loss of 40% of cells in Lewy body dementia renders the sufferers prone to develop drug-induced extrapyramidal syndromes.

Reference:

- Klockgether T (2004) Parkinson's disease: clinical aspects. *Cell and Tissue Research.* **318**(1): 115–20.

53 **True.**

Jerome Frank and others have emphasised various important factors in group therapy, such as *instillation of hope*. *Universality* comes into play when patients learn that others in the group may have had very similar experiences and feelings. *Vicarious learning* is where the patient benefits from other members' therapy experiences or models new future behaviours on the therapist or other patients.

Reference:

- Frank JD (1961) *Persuasion and Healing.* Johns Hopkins Press, Baltimore.

54 **True.**

In cue exposure the link between the stimulus (which triggers the unwanted behaviour) and the behaviour itself is weakened by allowing the stimulus to continue and preventing the usual response.

55 **False.**

Infants with phenylketonuria have similar minimal requirements of phenylalanine to normal children. Too severe a restriction can lead to tissue breakdown and rising levels of phenylalanine.

56 The grief process in families with a newly diagnosed child with learning disability may lead to 'shopping around' in families fixated at the 'grief' stage.

57 Huntington's disease is characterised by loss of alpha rhythms on EEG.

58 Males with schizophrenia (compared to females with schizophrenia) have fewer relapses.

59 Boys and girls who later go on to develop schizophrenia have the same levels of premorbid intellectual and social functioning.

60 In exhibitionism the offenders are characteristically over 50 years of age.

56 **True.**
'Shopping around' has been described by Professor Bicknell in families fixated at the denial stage. 'Bargaining' with professionals occurs before acceptance.

Reference:

- Bicknell J (1983) The psychopathology of handicap. *Br J Med Psychol.* **56**: 167–78.

57 **True.**
The EEG in Huntington's disease characteristically shows poorly developed or complete loss of alpha rhythms. The record may flatten as the disease progresses.

58 **False.**
Angermeyer *et al.* (1989) found that over an eight-year follow-up period men had a greater risk of re-admission and that their admissions tended to be much longer.

Reference:

- Angermeyer MC, Goldstein JM and Kuhn L (1989) Gender and the course of schizophrenia: differences in treated outcomes. *Schizophrenia Bull.* **10**: 430–59.

59 **False.**
Boys who go on to develop schizophrenia are more likely to have antecedent defects of intellectual and social functioning than girls. On CT and MRI brain scans there is evidence that males with schizophrenia more often have structural abnormalities of neurodevelopmental origin, including things like cysts of the septum pellucidum and obstetric complications.

Reference:

- Lewis S (1992) Sex and schizophrenia: vive la différence. *Br J Psychiatr.* **161**: 445–50.

60 **False.**

Exposure is the deliberate exposure of the genitalia by a man in the presence of an unwilling woman, where the man has no intention of progression to sexual intercourse. The majority of offenders are young men aged 15–25 years. Only 5% have mental retardation; 20% of offenders are 'sociopathic' and expose an erection for sadistic pleasure; their prognosis is worse.

Reference:

- Bancroft J (1989) *Human Sexuality and its Problems.* Churchill Livingstone, Edinburgh.

---

61 Shagreen patches are associated with tuberous sclerosis.

62 Cognitive analytic therapy does not involve work with the transference.

63 The oculovestibular response is helpful in diagnosing psychogenic coma.

64 Convulsions are associated with prolonged high-dose cocaine dependence.

65 In pregnancy benzodiazepines do not cross the placenta.

---

61 **True.**

Adenoma sebaceum, cafe-au-lait spots and shagreen patches occur in tuberous sclerosis.

62 **False.**

Cognitive analytic therapy (CAT) derives from the work of Anthony Ryle, who was a director of Sussex University's Health Service until 1979 and later became a consultant psychotherapist. The therapy work uses fairly classical concepts such as transference, interpretations and dream work associated with newer tools such as target problems, target problem procedures and sequential diagrammatic reformulations. In the latter the patient and therapist work out typical sequences of behaviour that the patient performs and often relates these to parental attributes.

63 **True.**

The oculovestibular response is abnormal in organic coma. A tonic response occurs in cortical lesions. An asymmetrical response suggests a focal brainstem lesion or a drug-induced coma. Absence of the response occurs in profound brainstem disturbance or drug overdose coma.

64 True.

65 False.
Benzodiazepines do cross the placenta and because the foetal liver metabolism is minimal benzodiazepines are concentrated in foetal tissues.

---

66 Most infants form attachments to several people.

67 School refusal exhibits several peak ages of presentation.

68 There is no geographical variation in the prevalence of conduct disorder.

69 Childhood hyperactivity and conduct disorder show equally strong prediction of adult antisocial personality disorder.

70 Cognitive behavioural psychotherapy is the psychological treatment of choice for children and adolescents with anxiety and depressive disorders.

---

66 True.
At 10 months 41% of infants have only one attachment but by 18 months only 13% had only one attachment. There appears to be a hierarchy of attachment objects with mother at the top.

Reference:

* Schaffer HR and Emerson PE (1964) The development of social attachments in infancy. *Monographs of Social Research in Child Development.* **29:** 94.

67 True.
There are three peaks of presentation for school refusal: approximately age 5 (start of primary school), age 11 (transition to secondary school) and age 14 onwards.

Reference:

* Goodman R and Scott S (eds) (2005) *Child Psychiatry.* Blackwell, Oxford.

68 False.
The diagnosis of conduct disorder is more prevalent in urban areas.

Reference:

* Rutter M *et al.* (1976) Adolescent turmoil: fact or fiction? *J Child Psychol Psychiatry.* **17:** 35–56.

69 **True.**

Reference:

- Simonoff E *et al.* (2004) Predictors of antisocial personality. *Br J Psych.* **184**: 118–27.

70 **True.**
From the available evidence CBT is the most effective psychological treatment for these internalising disorders.

Reference:

- Compton S *et al.* (2004) *Journal of the American Academy of Children and Adolescents Psychiatry.* **43**: 8.

---

71 The 'squiggle game' is used in the assessment of childhood dyslexia.

72 Loss of consciousness does not occur in complex partial seizures.

73 Intracerebral tumours are found in about 3% of adult patients presenting with complex partial seizures.

74 Gilles de la Tourette's syndrome usually presents initially with motor tics.

75 Obsessive compulsive disorder is less likely to respond to placebo than depression.

---

71 **False.**
The 'squiggle game' was devised by Winnicott as a way of getting into contact with the child. The clinician uses the drawings, the child's description of the squiggles and the child's approach to the game as a way of gaining some understanding of the child's concerns.

Reference:

- Winnicott D (1970) *Therapeutic Consultations in Child Psychiatry.* Hogarth Press, London.

72 **False.**
Complex partial seizures (CPS) are associated with impairment of consciousness and loss of consciousness can occur from the outset.

73 **False.**
Intracerebral tumours are found in about 10–15% of adult patients presenting with complex partial seizures.

74 True.
Motor tics of the head are the initial presentation at a mean age of seven years. Vocal tics may start around the age of 11, and coprolalia (which occurs in only 30% of patients) begins around the age of 13.

75 True.
A placebo response of 5% has been shown in OCD whereas depression enjoys a 30% placebo response rate.

---

76 The point prevalence for eating disorders in young British women is 20%.

77 Kluver-Bucy syndrome results from damage to subcortical areas of the brain.

78 Pick's disease is characterised by status spongiosus.

79 Ventricular dilatation out of proportion to sulcal atrophy is a feature of normal pressure hydrocephalus.

80 Immigrants who are refugees have a lower psychiatric morbidity than other kinds of immigrant because they have a positive view of their new surroundings.

---

76 False.
Prevalence rates in some studies of eating disorders may be artificially low since anorexic people avoid answering difficult questions on eating behaviour. A reliable point prevalence for broadly defined eating disorders in young British females is about 4–5%.

Reference:

• King MB (1989) Eating disorders in a general practice population: prevalence, characteristics and follow-up at 12–18 months. *Psychol Med.* **Suppl. 14.** Cambridge University Press, Cambridge.

77 True.
The Kluver-Bucy syndrome is associated with blunting of the emotions, agnosias, unrestrained exploring, an oral tendency with altered eating behaviour and hypersexuality.

78 False.
Status spongiosus is characteristic of Creutzfeldt-Jakob disease.

79 True.

80 **False.**
Rack suggested that there were three types of migrant: a gastarbeiter, or guest worker, who intends to return; an exile who migrates after political upheaval or natural disaster; and the settler who migrates with positive expectations. Refugees would count as 'exiles' in Rack's classification. Refugees have a particularly high psychiatric morbidity because of prior trauma which may cause post-traumatic stress disorder, or trigger affective illness or schizophrenia.

Reference:

• Rack PH (1986) Migration and mental illness. In: JL Cox (ed.) *Transcultural Psychiatry*. Croom Helm, London.

---

81 A split between a large managed group and a small supervisory group is a characteristic feature of a total institution according to Goffman (1961).

82 Linear causality is a phenomenon associated with systemic family therapy.

83 Erectile impotence occurs in 10% of 40-year-old males in the general population.

84 In an exploratory initial interview with a 12-year-old girl who has possibly been sexually abused an anatomically correct doll should be used.

85 Prominent language disorder in association with cognitive decline is a key feature of Huntington's disease.

---

81 **True.**
Total institutions like prisons, special hospitals, asylums and monasteries have all-encompassing tendencies. They break down the normal separations that we all enjoy between work, play and sleep, in that all activities are under the same authority in the same place. All activities are tightly scheduled and occur in the name of some rational plan according to the aims of the institution. There is a split between a large managed group (inmates/patients) and a small supervisory group (prison officers/nurses). Communication between inmates to higher staff levels (e.g. patients to doctors) is controlled (e.g. by nurses).

Reference:

• Goffman E (1961) *Asylums*. Harmondsworth, Penguin.

82 **False.**
Systems theory was described by von Bertalaffny in 1973. There are various features. *Homeostasis* is the mechanism where a system (family) in steady state will compensate for any change, or resist attempts to impose or create change. In families causality is circular not linear and elements such as feedback loops may operate.

Reference:

- von Bertalaffny L (1973) *General Systems Theory. Foundations, development, applications.* George Braziller, New York.

83 **False.**
Erectile impotence occurs in 1.9% of 40-year-olds.

Reference:

- Kinsey AC, Pomeroy WB and Martin CE (1948) *Sexual Behaviour in the Human Male.* Saunders, Philadelphia.

84 **False.**
An anatomically correct doll would be useful in an interview with a younger child; instead, art and drawing materials might be used, including more detailed anatomical drawing. By the age of 10 or 12, a child can be as proficient at recall as an adult.

Reference:

- Jones DPH and McQuiston MG (1988) *Interviewing the Sexually Abused Child.* Gaskell, London.

85 **False.**
Cognitive decline in the absence of language disorder is characteristic of Huntington's disease and suggests a sub-cortical origin for the dementia.

---

86 Epilepsy in Down's syndrome is no more prevalent than in the general population.

87 An early indicator of dementia in people with Down's syndrome is impairment of receptive language function.

88 Tricyclic antidepressants are considered potentially teratogenic in pregnancy.

89 Parents of autistic children are more likely to themselves have a *previous* history of anxiety disorder (than in the general population).

90 Phenylketonuria (PKU) is inherited in an autosomal recessive fashion.

86 **False.**
Seizures occur in about 7% of people with Down's syndrome.

Reference:

● Safstrom CE *et al.* (1991) Seizures in children with Down's syndrome: aetiology, characteristics and outcome. *Devel Med Child Neurol.* **33**: 191–200.

87 **True.**

Reference:

● Young EC and Kramer BM (1991) Characteristics of age-related language decline in adults with Down's syndrome. *Ment Retard.* **29**: 75–9.

88 **False.**
Tricyclic antidepressants are associated with case reports of birth difficulties in late pregnancy – neonates with CNS depression, respiratory acidosis, and convulsions.

89 **True.**
Twenty-four per cent of the parents of autistic children have anxiety disorders prior to the birth of the autistic child. Twelve per cent of fathers have Asperger's. The conversational language of parents of autistic children often has autistiform elements.

References:

● Gillberg C, Gillberg IC and Steffenburg S (1992) Siblings and parents of children with autism: a controlled population-based study. *Devel Med Child Neurol.* **34**: 389–98.
● Landa R *et al.* (1992) Social language use in parents of autistic individuals. *Psychol Med.* **22**: 245–54.

90 **True.**
The incidence range of PKU is 1 per 10 000 to 1 per 20 000 live births. PKU is inherited in an autosomal recessive fashion.

---

91 The neuropathological consequences of poisoning can be imaged on brain MRI.

92 Benzodiazepines produce an increase in fast beta activity on the EEG.

93 Clozapine interacts with warfarin.

94 Benzodiazepines increase stage 4 and REM sleep.

95 Typical features of right (non-dominant) parietal lobe damage include ipsilateral neglect in which the patient may ignore deficits on his right-hand side.

91 True.

Reference:

- Yudofsky SC and Hales RE (1997) *Textbook of Neuropsychiatry* (3e). American Psychiatric Press, Arlington, VA.

92 True.

93 True.
Clozapine is protein-bound, like warfarin, hence the interaction.

94 False.
Benzodiazepines decrease stage 4 and REM sleep and, following withdrawal, rebound REM with disturbed sleep may occur.

95 False.
Features of right (non-dominant) parietal lobe damage include contralateral neglect in which the patient may ignore deficits on his left-hand side.

---

96 Cocaine taking rapidly links reward with secondary cues.
97 A rating scale to measure the locus of control was introduced by Rotter (1966).
98 The majority of the body's stores of serotonin are within the central nervous system.
99 As clozapine has less affinity for D1 receptors than phenothiazines it causes fewer extrapyramidal side effects.
100 In cases of severe depression basal fasting serum growth hormone concentrations are greatly decreased.

---

96 True.
Cocaine taking rapidly links reward with secondary cues. These associated cues are very difficult to unlearn, so that environmental factors such as objects (like needles), people, occasions or places may trigger the association and cue cocaine abuse.

Reference:

- Strang J, Johns A and Caan W (1993) Cocaine in the UK. *Br J Psychiatr.* **162**: 1–13.

97 True.
Rotter (1966) introduced the concept of the internal locus of control where events, feelings and experiences are perceived as attributable to personal action. Where they are perceived as beyond personal responsibility this is an external locus of control.

Reference:

● Rotter JB (1966) Generalised expectancies for internal versus external control of re-inforcement. *Psychol Monogr.* 80: 609.

98 **False.**
Less than 2% of total body serotonin is in the CNS.

99 **True.**

100 **False.**

Extended Matching Items

Q1 Effective treatment strategies for antipsychotic-induced tardive dyskinesia include:

● ECT
● adding another antipsychotic
● using an alternative antipsychotic, e.g. quetiapine
● using adjunctive tetrabenazine
● withdrawing or reducing any coprescribed anticholinergic
● prescribing a calcium channel blocker, e.g. nifedipine
● a 'drug holiday'
● using the lowest effective dose long term.

A1 Effective treatment strategies for antipsychotic-induced tardive dyskinesia include:

● ECT	T
● adding another antipsychotic	F
● using an alternative antipsychotic, e.g. quetiapine	T
● using adjunctive tetrabenazine	T
● withdrawing or reducing any coprescribed anticholinergic	T
● prescribing a calcium channel blocker, e.g. nifedipine	T
● a 'drug holiday'	F
● using the lowest effective dose long term	T

People have used adjunctive treatments such as tetrabenazine, benzo-diazepines, buspirone, calcium antagonists or beta blockers. ECT can be helpful. So-called drug holidays appear to be detrimental and have been linked to relapse.

Reference:

● Bazire S (1995) *Psychotropic Drug Directory* (10e), p.105. Fivepin Ltd.

Q2 Therapeutic factors that Yalom found to be important in group psychotherapy include:

● projection
● cohesiveness
● universality
● altruism
● catharsis
● ambivalence
● splitting.

A2 Therapeutic factors that Yalom found to be important in group psychotherapy include:

● projection   F
● cohesiveness   T
● universality   T
● altruism   T
● catharsis   T
● ambivalence   F
● splitting   F

Highly cohesive groups have a better record of attendance, punctuality, activity by their members and stability (Yalom, 1975). Universality enables patients to see that other group members have similar experiences, difficulties and feelings to their own. Catharsis must be linked with insight to be helpful. Yalom *et al.* (1977) suggested that catharsis without an opportunity to integrate the emotional experience can have harmful effects.

References:

● Yalom ID (1975) *The Theory and Practice of Group Psychotherapy.* Basic Books, New York.
● Yalom ID *et al.* (1977) The impact of a weekend group experience on individual therapy. *Archives of General Psychiatry.* 34(4): 399–415.

MRCPsych Part II: Essay

Natasha Walford

Introduction

The essay paper is often the one that causes the greatest amount of anxiety in the MRCPsych written examination. For many of us it has been many years since we have had to write an essay, probably dating back to A-level exams where we had to regurgitate as many facts as possible in a seemingly very short space of time – a very unpleasant memory! Fortunately, in comparison to that, this paper is surprisingly straightforward.

The Royal College requirement for essay writing really reflects the importance placed on the ability to communicate in psychiatry. It requires the ability to communicate a balanced argument allowing the readers to reach their own conclusions – very similar to discussing treatment options with a patient in a clinic, which is something we all do every day.

What is an essay?

The word 'essay' itself can cause some confusion. The English dictionary says an essay is 'a short piece of prose writing on a specific topic'.

For those of us who find essay writing difficult, it should be comforting to note that the verb 'essay' means 'to attempt', being similar to the French verb 'essayer' meaning to try. Most essays are comprised of a written document held together in a structured way so the reader knows where it is heading.

College requirements

Candidates are required to write *one* essay from a choice of three during a one-and-a-half hour exam.

The College asks the candidates to *integrate* knowledge rather than regurgitate every fact they know and to organise the information to develop a reasoned argument. The College states that the information should be presented clearly and also that candidates should support their argument by using knowledge from relevant literature including:

- textbooks
- ICD-10/DSM-IV
- journals
- supporting evidence from your clinical experience and any audits and research that you have undertaken.

There has been a recent change in the examination – a good one! There is now only one essay that must be answered in contrast to previous exams where two were required. This removed the time restriction. Unlike in the old exam, there is now no division between general adult psychiatry and the psychiatric specialties and candidates should expect that all three questions will encompass aspects of general adult psychiatry and one or more of the different clinical specialties.

Read the questions properly

It is very important for candidates to read the questions properly. Even if you are in a panic and cannot answer any of the questions or alternatively if you are delighted that you see a familiar topic that you have rehearsed at home – STOP – and for goodness sake read the question again properly. For example, if the question says 'throughout the life cycle' it would be necessary for the candidate to consider the relevant aspects of the question from the perspective of childhood, adulthood and old age. A discussion about adult aspects only would lead to a poor mark even if more knowledge on adult aspects of the subject was documented than the entire knowledge of the examiners!

How are marks awarded?

Essays are marked out of ten:

1   extremely poor
2   very poor

3   poor
4   better but still a fail
5   borderline pass
6   pass
7   good pass
8   excellent
9   outstanding
10 doesn't happen.

Each essay is marked independently by two examiners. The mean mark is then awarded. Where there is a differential of greater than two marks (e.g. 3 and 6) the paper is re-marked.

What do I need to do to achieve a safe pass?

Firstly and perhaps most importantly write legibly.

1   *Illegibility will be penalised.*
It stands to reason that a tired examiner who is marking his fifteenth essay late into the night will be more amenable if he can read the work easily.

2   *Leave a space between each sentence.*
It helps if you leave a blank line between each sentence as this can make a jumbled essay easier on the eye and also enables any corrections or last minute amendments to be done neatly. Note that this is actually hard to remember to do if you have not practised writing essays in this manner.

3   *Writing style and fluency is important.*
Marks are also awarded for writing style, basic scientific knowledge and clinical knowledge, and extra marks will be awarded for references to relevant literature (*see* below).

4   *A good structure is necessary.*
Considering that the essay should be about 10 pages (double-spaced, one page written every 7–8 minutes), a good structure is very important.

An essay should start with an *introduction*. Why is this topic of interest? It is important to attract the attention of the examiner and entice them into actually wanting to read your essay. The opening statement should illustrate the relevance of the topic, how important it is to modern-day practice and should boost the College's ego for selecting such an interesting and stimulating essay title.

Your *argument* is the main body of the essay. Even if you have very strong views about the topic do not just write about how much you disagree with it as your examiner might have opposing views. For example, if the essay is

'Discuss the statement that lithium has a limited role in the modern-day management of female bipolar affective disorder', it would not go down well if you wrote 10 pages on the negatives of lithium when the examiner marking the paper uses it as first-line treatment in all his patients and has just written a paper on how useful a drug it is. A balanced argument is the key to a good essay.

It is up to each individual to set out his or her own argument. Some like to organise their essay into two parts. Using the above example they would first summarise all their points in favour of lithium and in part two discuss all the arguments against lithium. The other way is to argue each point as you go along. For example, you could start by referring to the NICE (National Institute for Health and Clinical Excellence) guidelines that lithium is still the number one mood stabiliser in the United Kingdom due to its effectiveness in clinical trials but then argue that it is difficult to use in acute episodes as patients are often too ill to consent to treatment, and mention the risk of relapse if medication is suddenly stopped. This theme could be continued throughout the essay and then summed up in the conclusion. There is no right or wrong way. Personally I prefer the first method as I can focus initially on why lithium is a brilliant drug and write down everything I think is great about it and then I can stop and think of all the bad points. If you use the first method, it is always important to leave a space in the first section, as you will think of some additional points as you start to argue against it.

The *conclusion* should some sum up the evidence and ideally you should come down on one side and support this with your reasons.

5   *Do use a plan.*

To make your argument go as smoothly as possible a plan is always a really good idea. It is also useful to keep it on your finished paper so that the examiner before reading the essay will know in which direction it is going. It will provide you with an opportunity to brainstorm ideas as well. It will also help you to find out at an early stage if you have enough ideas to complete an essay on your choice of title and may in fact lead to you changing essays. It is much better to do this at the start rather than when you are on page three of your essay and half an hour into the exam.

Easy tips

OK, that is the scary bit out of the way. There are ways to make this paper much more straightforward and a very easy way to make up for marks lost on the very much hit-or-miss MCQ paper (I did not enjoy that paper!).

From personal experience the best advice I can give is to try to spot the title before you get into the examination. Now, I do not mean trying to hack into the College computer system to preview the exam paper. There are several legal ways you can help yourself with this paper.

1   Certain topics are common and tend to be repeated – look at websites with past titles, for example 'the superego café', 'the Royal College website', suggestions from recent revision courses, e.g. the Manchester course.
2   Read the recent articles in the Yellow Journal. Look at topical articles and plan essays on these topics. Form study groups with your friends and each write some essay plans and then meet and share ideas.
3   List the recent topical subjects, e.g. early intervention in psychosis, and learn the names of people who have published work in this field. The year of publication is not particularly important. Remember that it is general psychiatrists who are marking these papers. They will not know the year and month the article was published and will not have time to check, but they will be aware of the major names in each field.

Do not be put off by the question itself. It is often very distressing when you have prepared and memorised brilliant essays for the topics you predicted would be in the exam and none of them has come up or they have but the question is of no relevance to the answer you prepared on the topic. I am sure this scenario sounds very familiar to many doctors who have sat the exam.
   DON'T PANIC!
   First, re-read all the questions. Look at the topic in the broadest sense first and then focus in on constitutional issues.
   In my exam (Autumn 2003) the titles were:

1   Psychotherapeutic approaches should be considered in the care of older adults with mental health problems. Discuss this statement critically with reference to the range and efficacy of psychological treatments in the elderly.
2   You are asked to brief your service manager on the factors involved in prolonging inpatient stays on an acute admissions ward. Outline your response and suggest how these problems could be tackled.
3   Describe the criteria that a new syndrome would need to satisfy in order to be added to the classification system of psychiatric disorders. Illustrate your answer with particular reference to post-traumatic stress disorder and social phobia.

I read them once, then twice and then again. I had done lots of essay plans, even written out whole essays, but none of the above options seemed remotely enticing – the exit doors were now staring at me!

I stayed in the exam and read the questions again. I had written a full essay on the evidence base for CBT – it was really good (if I say so myself) but it did not have any evidence for CBT in the elderly. Maybe there had been no work done in this age group but I did not know and had not bothered to find out – old age psychiatry was not my thing!

All I could think about essay number two was that hospitals need more beds and I had stopped reading the third choice as it was definitely a no-go zone. In fact if I had calmed down and attempted number two I could have written a very good essay but I opted for number one and wrote broadly about how the elderly should not be discriminated against for psychological treatments because of their age and wrote about the efficacy of CBT, psychotherapy and counselling in general. I passed with this essay.

Number two really was much more straightforward and shows that thinking broadly about the topic initially and then focusing on key areas can be a useful technique. A plan for essay number two could include:

Introduction – In general discuss the problem of bed shortages, especially in inner-city areas. Discuss how poorly patients have to be admitted out of area because beds are blocked by accommodation issues and lack of community staff.

In the *body of the essay* write about the factors prolonging stay.

1 Long duration of untreated psychosis before presentation therefore making psychosis more resistant to treatment (*see* Richard Drake's paper below under 'Schizophrenia').
2 Talk about better education for GPs, development of early intervention services, availability of more psychologists for insight work, CBT, etc.
3 The problem of substance misuse in this population aggravating psychiatric conditions which could be helped by better public education and more funding for substance misuse services.
4 Problems of high expressed emotion in families and the need for more education and support for carers and relatives.
5 The problem of finding suitable accommodation for inpatients and the lack of funding available for after-services like rehab and supported accommodation.
6 Staff shortages for crisis teams, CMHTs (community mental health teams), day hospitals, drop-in centres – all these services have been shown to prevent relapse and decrease the need for hospital admissions but the money is not available.
7 Stigma of psychiatric illness – people not wanting to take medications for fear of being labelled psychiatrically unwell – combat by better public education.

8   Side effects of medications – doctors and nurses should be asking about embarrassing side effects, including sexual ones that may not be volunteered.

The points are endless.

References to literature

Reference to literature is important. It is not expected that candidates know the year, month and exact journal in which the article was published, as the marking doctors probably will not know either. However, what is important is to show that you have read the latest pieces of research and are using the information to guide your practice. What I found useful was to learn the main names in common areas so that I could demonstrate some knowledge of recent articles in a field even if I had not read the papers in question.

List of common references

Eating disorders

- Dare C, Eisler I, Russel G, Treasure J and Dodge L (2001) Psychological therapies for adults with anorexia nervosa: randomized controlled trial of outpatients treatments. *British Journal of Psychiatry.* **178**: 216–21. (NB: This is the paper that led to the only category B recommendation in the NICE guidelines advocating family therapy for young anorexics.)

Other important names in eating disorder research include S Gowers who wrote a paper concluding that if possible it is better to treat anorexics as outpatients as they have a better prognosis than inpatients.

- Gowers S, Weetman J, Shore A, Hossain F and Elvins R (2000) Impact of hospitalization on the outcome of adolescent anorexia nervosa. *British Journal of Psychiatry.* **176**(2): 138–41.

Janet Treasure, Consultant at the Maudsley, has also written books to help guide our practice.

- Schmidt U, Treasure J and Treasure T (1993) *Getting Better Bit(e) by Bit(e): a survival kit for sufferers of bulimia and binge eating disorders.* Psychology Press, London.

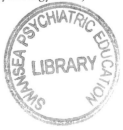

Schizophrenia

Important research names include Shon Lewis who has done a lot of work into early detection and intervention of psychosis using cognitive behavioural therapy versus treatment as normal in young adults deemed at high risk of developing psychosis.

- Larsen T, Friis S, Haahr U *et al*. (2001) Early detection and intervention in first episode schizophrenia: a critical review. *Acta Psychiatrica Scandinavica*. **103**: 323–34.
- Morrison A, French P, Walford L, Lewis S, Kilcommons A, Green J, Parker S and Bentall R (2004) Cognitive therapy for the prevention of psychosis in people at ultra-high risk. Randomised control trial. *Br J Psychiatrists*. **185**(4): 291–7.
- Warner R (2001) Combating the stigma of schizophrenia. *Epidemiologia Psychiatria Sociale*. **10**: 12–17.

In terms of treating psychosis, the longer the delay in treatment, the worse the prognosis (duration of untreated psychosis), summarised in a paper by Richard Drake *et al*. in 2000.

- Drake R, Haley C, Akhtar S and Lewis S (2000) Causes and consequences of duration of untreated psychosis in schizophrenia. *British Journal of Psychiatry*. **177**: 511–15.
- Vaughan and Leff (1985) *Expressed Emotion in Families: its significance for mental illness*. Guilford Press, London.

Cannabis

Studies involving the Duneadin population have shown that the younger people use cannabis, the greater the chance of developing psychosis.

- Arseneault L, Cannon M, Poulton R, Murray R, Caspi A and Moffitt T (2002) Cannabis use in adolescence and risk for adult psychosis: longitudinal prospective study. *BMJ*. **325**: 1212–13.

Perhaps the first informative paper on the use of cannabis and the development of psychosis was Zammit *et al*. (2002).

- Patton G, Coffey C, Carlin J, Degenhardt L, Lynskey M and Hall W (2002) Cannabis use and mental health in young people: cohort study. *BMJ*. **325**: 1195–8.
- Zammit S, Allebeck P *et al*. (2002) Self reported cannabis use as a risk factor for schizophrenia in Swedish conscripts of 1969: historical cohort study. *BMJ*. **325**: 1199.

Suicide

Key names include Louis Appleby and Keith Hawton who have both done a lot of work into the risk factors for suicide.

- Appleby L, Shaw J, Amos T *et al*. (1999) *Safer Services. Report of the National Confidential Inquiry into Suicides and Homicides by People with Mental Illness*. Stationery Office, London.
- Barraclough B *et al*. (1974) A hundred cases of suicide: clinical aspects. *British Journal of Psychiatry*. **125**: 355–73.
- Hawton K, Townsend E, Arensman E and Gunnell D (2001) Psychosocial and pharmacological treatments for deliberate self harm. *The Cochrane Library*, Vol. 2. Update Software, Oxford.

Mood disorders

- Brown GW and Harris T (1990) *Social Origins of Depression*. Routledge, London.
- Burgess S, Geddes J, Hawton K, Townsend E, Jamison K and Goodwin G (2001) Lithium for maintenance treatment of mood disorders. *Cochrane Library*, Vol. 3. Update Software, Oxford.
- Coppen A *et al*. (1967) Tryptophan in the treatment of depression. *The Lancet*. 2(7527): ii 78–80.
- Goodnick P, Chaudry T, Artadi J (2000) Women's issues in mood disorders. *Expert Opinions in Psychotherapy*. **1**: 903–16.
- Sachs G, Koslow C and Ghaemi S (2000) The treatment of bipolar depression. *Bipolar Disorders*. **2**: 256–60.
- Schildkraut JI (1967) The catecholamine hypothesis of affective disorders. *Int J of Psychiatry*. 4(3): 203–17.

This can be done for all the major topics that could come up in the exam so even if the question totally throws you, you can at least reel off some important names and papers in that field.

I have included at the end of this chapter the last few Royal College Essay papers as examples to see how questions are typically phrased.

For those of you that are re-sitting the exam it may help to know that in a few years the MRCPsych examinations as we know them will be abolished to keep in line with Europe and the new junior training scheme. Instead, there will be a module-type assessment schedule where trainees would be constantly assessed throughout their training, and assessments will count towards becoming a member of the college.

To all of you who have worked really hard to pass the MRCPsych, the College offers a comforting statement: 'At least you will have the self-satisfaction that you actually passed the exam.'

Example essay questions

Set A

1   How does the presentation, assessment and treatment of depression differ in children and adolescents compared to adults? Discuss the implications of all the differences.
2   How would you organise high-quality psychiatric services for the mentally disordered on remand and serving sentences in prisons? How would you minimise suicide risks?
3   Discuss the pharmacological and psychological treatment of eating disorders and the implication for primary and secondary care services.

Set B

1   'There is no association between severe and enduring mental illness, physical ill health and social disadvantage.' Discuss in relation to psychotic illnesses.
2   Gender has no relevance in psychiatric illness. Discuss this with specific reference to mood and substance misuse disorders.
3   Harm reduction and abstinence targeted treatments are both used in the treatment of a range of addictive disorders. Discuss the relative advantages and disadvantages of each approach.

Set C

1   'Treatment-resistant depression can only be treated by biological methods and this treatment should only be provided by tertiary services.' Discuss this critically with reference to the evidence base.
2   'Early intervention in schizophrenia is critical for good long-term outcome.' Discuss this assertion and outline its implications for the provision of psychiatric services.
3   Discuss the relationship between adverse childhood experience and the later development of psychiatric illness with particular reference to personality disorders and affective disorders.

Set D

1   Discuss the ethical problems associated with mental health legislation, giving specific examples.
2   Discuss the optimum use of psychological treatment in schizophrenia and affective disorders with support from literature evidence.
3   Discuss the evidence base for the use of atypical neuroleptics in *first-onset* schizophrenia with support from literature evidence.

MRCPsych Part II: Critical Review Paper

Chris McWilliams

The Part II MRCPsych Examination underwent a major change in the Spring of 1999 when the Short Answer Question paper (SAQ) was replaced with the Critical Review Paper (CRP). This has also coincided with withdrawal of the research option due to lack of interest. Reasons for the change and the aims of the paper have been summarised in the *Psychiatric Bulletin* (1997) but it appears that the main reasons for change were:

- Analysis of results showed consistently that candidates' marks in the SAQ and Multiple-Choice Question (MCQ) papers correlated closely and assessed the same type of skills.
- Stress on the importance of evidence-based medicine to clinical practice requires that psychiatrists develop and maintain the necessary skills to critically assess published literature in terms of its scientific merit and relevance to clinical practice, research and audit. This is not tested elsewhere in the exam.

The Royal College of Psychiatrists has produced an information pack on the CRP where the aims of the Critical Review Paper are clearly stated. This also contains sample questions and should be required reading for candidates.

The main aims of introducing such a paper in terms of promoting various skills are summarised here.

1 Understanding research methodology and study design.
2 Understanding sources of problems and bias and detection of errors in research methodology.
3 Understanding basic statistics.
4 Definitions of basic statistical measures, e.g. sensitivity, specificity, odds ratio.
5 Knowledge of methodology of systematic reviews and meta-analysis.
6 Determination of reliability and validity of research.

7 Evaluation of clinical relevance of research findings and their effects on clinical practice. Understanding how to detect errors in research methodology and design.

8 Understanding the process of the critical appraisal of a scientific paper.

9 Use of research data to generate further experiments which would confirm hypotheses or increase understanding.

10 Applying scientific results in an appropriate context to clinical practice.

The paper itself

This comprises the first part of the written paper and is allocated 90 minutes. It consists of an abridged version of a paper that has actually appeared in the scientific literature after being subject to peer review. Questions will depend on the nature of the paper but will refer to aspects of methodology, statistics, assessment of data and clinical relevance. Marks allocated to each question will be shown and length of answer suggested by spacing lines on the answer sheet. Marking will be conducted as for the old SAQ, i.e. by two separate examiners using a model answer provided by the college question setter.

Sample paper and model answer

- Dehlin O, Rubin B, Rundgren Å (1995) Double-blind comparison of zopiclone and flunitrazepam in elderly insomniacs with special focus on residual effects. *Curr Med Res Opin.* **13**: 317–24.

Introduction

Subjective sleep quality becomes very much impaired in older age groups and this is also reflected in an increased hypnotic drug consumption in old age.

Benzodiazepines are widely used as hypnotics for older people and the side-effects of such drugs are also well-known. One of the most distressing side-effects of benzodiazepines with a medium or long elimination half-life is a residual effect the following day, commonly known as hangover. Drugs with a shorter elimination half-life could therefore benefit older people by providing sleep without residual effects the next day.

Zopiclone is a hypnotic compound belonging to the cyclopyrrolone group, non-related to the benzodiazepines, but with a similar activity and equal efficacy in insomnia. Zopiclone is rapidly absorbed and has a plasma elimination half-life of 4–5 hours in young subjects, increased to ~6 h in patients over 65 years old and to ~8 h in those over 80 years of age. However, this is unlikely to have a profound clinical significance. There are no clinically significant active metabolites.

Flunitrazepam is commonly prescribed to treat insomnia in elderly patients. This benzodiazepine has a fairly long elimination half-life, 13–19 h, which could contribute to hangover effects during the daytime.

This study compared a low dose of zopiclone, 5 mg, and the commonly used dose of flunitrazepam, 1 mg, with its focus on efficacy (quality of sleep) and on residual effects in elderly patients with insomnia. The hypothesis was that the clinical efficacy of the low dose of 5 mg zopiclone should be as efficacious as 1 mg of flunitrazepam but with less influence on alertness.

Methods and materials

In a multicentre, double-blind, randomized, parallel group study performed at 10 geriatric clinics in Sweden, patients of both sexes over 60 years of age were invited to take part. They had to be in a stable medical condition suffering from insomnia of at least 1 month's duration with a need for hypnotic treatment according to the investigator's judgement. The patients were to be intellectually fit to understand and follow simple instructions. To be included, they had to score ≥24 points on the MMSE, i.e. the Mini-Mental State Examination. Both previously treated and untreated patients were included. At least two of the following criteria had to be fulfilled to be included:

1   Latency of sleep onset more than 30 min.
2   More than two awakenings each night.
3   Time taken to go back to sleep after nocturnal awakening of more than 45 min.
4   Less than 6 h of sleep each night ≤80% of desired sleep time.
5   Morning awakening at least 2 h before expected time.

Exclusion criteria were patients who were suffering from insomnia due to severe somatic or psychotic diseases; with myasthenia gravis; with known severe liver or renal insufficiency; suffering from the sleep apnoea syndrome; with known allergy to benzodiazepines or zopiclone; undergoing neuroleptic and/or antidepressant treatment; with alcohol or drug abuse.

Each patient received the following treatment regimen:

● Week 1 (4–7 nights): each night one placebo capsule.
● Weeks 2–3: each night one 5 mg zopiclone capsule (zopiclone group) or one 1 mg flunitrazepam capsule (flunitrazepam group).
● Week 4: each night one placebo capsule.

The beginning and end of the study were single-blinded with the investigators knowing about the placebo treatment.

Efficacy variables

In a patient diary the following variables were recorded daily by the patient:

- Morning notes (30 min after awakening):
  - How did you sleep last night? (visual analogue scale (VAS): extremely well – extremely badly).
  - How many times did you wake up? (number).
  - Did you wake up too early without being able to go back to sleep? (yes/no).
  - How did you feel on awakening? (VAS: extremely alert – extremely sleepy).
  - How easily did you wake up? (VAS: very easily – with extreme difficulty).
  - Do you feel rested? (VAS: totally – not at all).
  - Did you have difficulty in falling asleep? (VAS: extremely – not at all).
  - Do you remember having dreamt last night? (VAS: intensely – not at all).
  - If you remember a dream, was it unpleasant, neutral, pleasant?
- Evening notes (just after intake of the hypnotic):
  - State of calmness (VAS: very calm – very nervous; very relaxed – very tense).
  - Alertness during the day (VAS: extremely alert – extremely sleepy).
  - Need for daytime naps? (5-grade Likert scale).

Clinical assessments were done once a week by the investigators during the entire trial, and the following question was asked: 'How do you judge your sleep for the preceding week?'. Compliance was checked by the patient's response to the diary question: 'Did you take your sleeping pill last night?', and also by counting the pills at the visits to the doctor. A nurse checked that the patient complied with the instructions.

Safety variables

At all visits the investigator put the open-ended question: 'Have you noticed anything special?'. The answers were noted in the case report form. These were any events, positive or negative, that the subject experienced during the study. Adverse effects or intercurrent illness were considered as study events. The subject was asked the following non-specific question: 'How have you been feeling since your last visit?'.

Patients

A total of 107 patients entered the study and five dropped out during the 4 week period because they did not want to continue with the study. According to the protocol they could do so without giving any reason for their decision. The data shown is thus based on the 102 patients who completed the study. Fifty patients, 13 men and 37 women, completed their treatment in the zopiclone group; and 52, 17 men and 35 women, in the flunitrazepam group. They did not differ significantly in age (mean age 79 years, range 60–95 years) or body weight. Nor was there any difference in the length of history of insomnia between the groups (mean 10 years, range 1–60 years).

The MMSE showed no significant differences between the groups: the zopiclone group had a mean of 27.5 ± 2.5 SD points and the flunitrazepam group 27.8 ± 2.6 SD points.

Almost all patients suffered from conditions for which they took drugs other than hypnotics. Drugs known to interfere with sleep such as broncho-dilators, diuretics, beta-blockers, analgesics and antihistamines were evenly distributed between the groups.

The patients' main diagnoses are shown in Table I.

Table I: Main diagnoses of the patients

Diagnosis	Zopiclone group	Flunitrazepam group
Stroke	11	14
Other neurological disease	2	4
Fracture	7	4
Diabetes mellitus	3	1
Other disease	27	29

Statistics

All patients completing the study were included in the efficacy analysis. The analyses were made using the mean of the measurements recorded during each week. The treatment effect, calculated as the difference between week 1 and weeks 2 and 3, respectively, was analysed for each variable. The difference between the two treatments was tested using analysis of variance. p-Values below 0.05 were considered statistically significant.

Information and consent

The study was approved by the ethics committee of the University of Gothenburg prior to commencement and all patients gave their informed consent. The study was performed according to the Declaration of Helsinki (Tokyo Amendment).

Results

All patients tolerated both drugs well. The five drop-outs were not due to side-effects but to a wish from the patients to withdraw, and they gave no reason for their decision. A statistically significant difference between the treatments in difficulty falling asleep was noted in the data for weeks 2 and 3 (Table II).

Table II: Means and standard deviations (SD) and differences (p-values) in sleep parameters between zopiclone (Zopiclo) and funitrazepam (Flunitra) during the 2 weeks of active treatment

	Week 2 (1. week of active treatment)				
	Zopiclo	Zopiclo	Flunitra	Flunitra	
	Mean	SD	Mean	SD	p
How did you sleep last night?	30.7	15.8	27.0	20.6	0.08
How many times did you wake up?	1.36	0.7	1.38	1.0	0.36
Did you wake up too early without being able to go back to sleep?	0.31	0.31	0.25	0.35	0.42
How did you feel on awakening?	31.4	18.4	33.2	22.6	0.65
How easily did you wake up?	42.3	19.1	45.4	25.0	0.73
Do you feel rested?	38.4	19.5	44.3	22.9	0.38
Did you have difficulty in falling asleep?	28.9	19.4	23.2	17.2	0.04
Do you remember having dreamt last night?	75.9	20.0	71.9	24.9	0.22
If you remember a dream, was it unpleasant, neutral, pleasant?	41.7	18.7	45.3	23.3	0.06
State of calmness	29.8	19.6	31.4	24.8	0.42
Alertness during the day	31.7	20.4	33.0	23.1	0.55
Need for daytime naps	2.8	0.7	2.9	0.7	0.87

	Week 3 (2. week of active treatment)				
	Zopiclo	Zopiclo	Flunitra	Flunitra	
	Mean	SD	Mean	SD	p
How did you sleep last night	35.5	21.4	30.8	20.2	0.09
How many times did you wake up?	1.58	0.92	1.49	1.17	0.08
Did you wake up too early without being able to go back to sleep?	0.30	0.33	0.29	0.34	0.77
How did you feel on awakening?	32.2	21.2	29.6	19.0	0.78
How easily did you wake up?	44.1	23.5	41.7	20.5	0.40
Do you feel rested?	40.2	22.8	40.5	20.4	0.93
Did you have difficulty in falling asleep?	34.6	22.7	24.2	18.5	0.002
Do you remember having dreamt last night?	76.1	22.5	70.9	25.3	0.55
If you remember a dream, was it unpleasant, neutral, pleasant?	45.9	21.5	42.7	18.5	0.83
State of calmness	33.1	22.8	30.1	23.0	0.97
Alertness during the day	33.8	22.6	32.1	23.0	0.69
Need for daytime naps	2.9	0.7	2.7	0.7	0.44

There was no significant difference in compliance ('Did you take your sleeping pill last night?') between the groups for any week, nor for the questions 'Have you noticed anything special?' and 'How have you been feeling since your last visit?'.

No serious or unexpected adverse events occurred and no patient dropped out due to adverse effects. The numbers of adverse effects experienced during the four weeks are shown in Table III. The type of adverse effects reported for three or more patients on either drug during weeks 2 and 3 together, as well as for the initial and final placebo week, are shown in Table IV.

Table III: Number of adverse effects experienced during the 4 weeks in the two treatment groups

Week	Zopiclone group	Flunitrazepam group
1 Placebo	23	34
2 Active treatment	24	30
3 Active treatment	23	23
4 Placebo	15	18

Table IV: Type of adverse effect (number of patients) reported in three or more patients on either drug during weeks 2 and 3 combined (active treatment) and during the initial and final placebo weeks

Symptom	Zopiclone	Flunitrazepam	Initial placebo week	Final placebo week
Vertigo	10	4	3	5
Depression	7	10	6	3
Arthralgia	7	5	6	0
Diarrhoea	2	6	0	0
Headache	2	6	8	3
Vomiting	0	0	9	3
Dry mouth	0	0	0	3
Myalgia	0	0	0	3
Vision problems	0	0	0	3

Question 1 (Background)

a) What is the clinical significance of the phenomenon described as 'hangover' in elderly patients?
b) How does the pharmacological profile of the two drugs in the study differ in their capacity to produce this effect?
c) How does the presence of clinically active metabolites prolong the action of a drug? Give three examples that may influence prescribing in psychiatry.

Answer 1 (Background)

a) Hypnotic medication is one of the most commonly prescribed groups of drugs in the elderly in hospital and in the community. Over-sedation is a common cause of comorbidity. The effects of many hypnotic drugs often persist into the following day. Common effects are acute and chronic confusional states, dizziness and falls. Misdiagnosis of dementia or depression may occur if a careful drug history is not taken. Problems of drug metabolism and elimination in the elderly render them much more susceptible to such problems than younger people.

b)   The main difference is in the elimination half-lives of the two drugs. Zopiclone has a relatively much shorter half-life and as such is likely to be eliminated from the body more quickly, reducing the capacity for producing 'hangover'.

c)   The effect is to prolong the effect of the drug by increasing elimination time. The time taken to eliminate the metabolite(s) is added to that of the parent compound. In addition if more drug is taken before elimination is complete then levels are liable to accumulate reaching toxic levels. The following drugs all have metabolites with significantly long half-lives:

- fluoxetine – norfluoxetine
- diazepam – desmethyldiazepam
- chlordiazepoxide – desmethylchlordiazepoxide
- lofepramine – desipramine.

Question 2 (Methodology)

a)   What are the main advantages of a double-blind placebo trial in this type of study?

b)   Outline briefly three potential sources of error or bias in this particular study.

c)   How would you assess the validity of a therapeutic trial?

d)   Given the above, how valid is this study?

e)   Why is it important to record adverse events in this type of trial?

Answer 2 (Methodology)

a)   A double-blind trial if properly conducted removes two potential areas of bias in ratings, i.e. those produced by the expectations of patients and raters.

b)   The study was conducted in many different centres, increasing the potential for the results to be scattered. The authors do not state whether the patients were hospitalised or in the community. There is no attempt to standardise sleeping conditions, i.e. did the patients sleep alone, with their partners or in dormitories? The patients have a considerable degree of physical illness – does this affect sleep? The study relies on self-rating only, a notoriously unreliable method in sleep assessment.

c)   Validity determines whether the study actually tests what it sets out to do. In therapeutic trials standard diagnoses, standard treatments and standard rating scales should be used. Inclusion and exclusion criteria should be clearly defined and adhered to. Randomisation and double blindness must be correctly carried out. Treatment groups must be clinically and demographically similar. A power calculation may be useful to indicate the size of study required to achieve a reasonable chance of obtaining a statistically significant result.

d)   The two groups are demographically and clinically similar and standard rating scales have been used. Some doubt must be expressed as to the use of self-rating scales and to the inclusion of such a clinically hetero-geneous group of patients. The study appears small and only achieves statistical significance on two parameters. There appears to be no problem with randomisation or double blindness. The study should be taken as having limited validity only.

e)   Adverse events occur in all drugs and are a frequent finding in the placebo treatment group. Reporting of adverse events is essential in order to determine the statistical significance of any excess of events caused by drug rather than placebo. Some indication of the severity of adverse events can be determined by the discontinuation rates due to adverse events at each stage.

Question 3 (Results)

a)   What do the results tell us about the relative comparability of the two groups?

b)   What are the chi-squared test and p values? What value of p is normally used to indicate whether a result has achieved signifi-cance?

c)   List all the results from Table II which achieve statistical signifi-cance. What is the difference between statistical and clinical sig-nificance?

d)   Comment on the side effects found in the placebo group.

Answer 3 (Results)

a)   Given the data provided it appears the two groups are clinically and demographically similar enough for valid comparisons to be made.

b)   The chi-squared test is a measure of statistical significance used to compare variables between two or more independent data sets. It uses the concept of the null hypothesis, i.e. that the variables are equally distributed between the groups. The test compares the differences between the findings of the study and those which would be expected if the null hypothesis were true. Statistical significance is expressed as a value of p, usually as a decimal (e.g. p=0.2 or as a percentage 20%). Most studies take a p value of 0.05 (5%) and below to denote statistical significance. Clinical significance may or may not be present at the same time. This is a much more subjective term and refers to whether a result would be sufficiently noticeable in a clinical setting to influence practice.
c)   The only result to achieve significance is that difficulty in falling asleep was less in the flunitrazepam group at weeks 2 and 3.
d)   Side effects are commonly found in placebo studies and often relate to gastrointestinal and neuropsychological complaints. The nature and frequency of the side effects noted in the placebo group is unremarkable given the demographic and clinical composition of the sample.

Question 4 (Discussion)

a)   List four ways you might arrange such a study to provide more meaningful data.
b)   Discuss the clinical relevance of the study.

Answer 4 (Discussion)

a)   Larger patient cohort. Choose patients with less co-existing physical illness. Use observer-rating scales. Control for sleeping environment.
b)   This study must be considered to be of only limited clinical use. The actual clinical status of the patients is poorly described. We do not know about the differences between drugs in different clinical or social settings and only small differences are noted in the results. There is no data to help determine choice of drug in clinical practice.

Improving performance in the CRP

The CRP presents a new challenge to trainee psychiatrists and their tutors who now have to ensure competence in reading and interpreting research and review papers and case reports. Candidates should ensure that they are up to date with significant studies in the Yellow Journal and practise presenting the findings. Books of CRP exercises are sure to appear shortly.

As with the rest of the exam, practice is the key. Journal clubs can be a useful forum for this and should be used effectively. Reading journals with the summary removed, then summarising the article oneself, is an especially valuable exercise. Candidates should also be aware of definition and application of various statistical tests as for the old SAQ and familiarise themselves with the principles behind evidence-based medicine as applied to psychiatry.

Suggested reading list

- Brown T and Wilkinson G (eds) (1999) *Critical Reviews in Psychiatry*. Royal College of Psychiatrists Seminar Series. Gaskell, London.
- Geddes J and Harrison P (1997) Evidence based psychiatry. Closing the gap between research and practice. *Br J Psych*. 171: 220–5.
- Royal College of Psychiatrists (1997) Proposed Critical Review Paper. *Psychiatric Bulletin*. 21: 381–2.
- Sackett D, Richardson W, Rosenburg W *et al.* (1996) *Evidence Based Medicine. How to teach evidence based medicine*. Churchill Livingstone, London.

It is also worth reading regularly *Evidence Based Medicine* and *Evidence Based Mental Health*, published by the BMJ.

The Cochrane Library is available to libraries on CD-ROM and the Cochrane Review Methodology database periodically updates information on research methodology.

MRCPsych Part II: Clinical Examinations

Introduction

In the MRCPsych Part II Clinical Examination the candidate will have to interview a carefully chosen patient at length and then present that patient to two examiners, demonstrating clinical skills and an ability to make a good differential diagnosis, but will also be expected to be fully conversant with management issues and prognosis.

The reason for failure of the Clinical Examination cannot be laid at the patient's or examiner's door. The fault can only lie in the candidate's preparation, presentation and discussion of the case.

To increase the chance of passing the Clinical Examination, the candidate must have considerable experience in presenting patients in an examination-like setting, and be confident enough to overcome any anxiety.

There are three rules: rehearsal, rehearsal and rehearsal.

Preparation

In the context of a busy service, the candidate must make time for a formal rehearsal at least once a week for two or three months before the examination. The prerequisites of a good session are as follows.

- The patient is new to the candidate.
- The session is devoted to examination rehearsal.
- The time spent both with the patient and the examiner is as near to the examination format as it can be.
- The examiner asks probing questions.
- The examiner is truthful and constructive in feedback.
- The session should be formalised to the extent that it may reproduce a mild degree of anxiety for the candidate.

The ideal session is very difficult to come by in real life. However, approximations can be achieved through:

- formal presentations in ward rounds
- peer syndicates being arranged locally in which potential candidates present cases to each other
- video presentations.

General points

The Clinical Examination and Patient Management Problems are usually held at the same centre on the same day. The day is long enough and stressful enough without the difficulty of getting all the way from home to the centre by car or train that day. Arrive the day before and stay overnight in a nearby hotel. Stay in comfort and treat yourself well! Eat a hearty breakfast! Dress comfortably so as to look confident, but also dress smartly and soberly. Dark, conservative colours are the order of the day. Try to look 'consultoid', and be comfortable in that attire.

Constructing the presentation

Most medical cases are formally presented by working through a list of headings. Psychiatric cases are no exception. The potential candidate will be familiar with the order of assessment and presentation, given here in Box 2 (for the sake of brevity, detail is omitted).

Box 2   The order of assessment

Reason for referral
Complaints
Present illness
Family history
Personal history:
- development
- medical/psychiatric
- forensic
- alcohol/drugs

Personality
Mental state:
- appearance and behaviour
- talk
- mood
- thought
- abnormal experiences
- insight
Cognitive examination

From the information elicited under each of these headings, the candidate constructs a differential diagnosis, or this is what is supposed to happen. In fact, usually somewhere halfway through the 'present complaint', the psychiatrist has generated preliminary diagnoses. During the rest of the interview, many of the questions will be asked in order to substantiate this.

Consequently, when presenting the case, the examinee should present it so that data under each of the relevant headings substantiates the differential diagnosis that he or she comes out with at the end. During the presentation of the case, it is of course important to emphasise these cardinal features.

The case may not be clear cut in that there is data substantiating more than one diagnosis. This must not be seen as a problem but as an interesting area of debate to present to the examiners. In this particular situation, the evidence supporting one diagnosis is balanced against the evidence supporting the other. As is recognised by most classification systems, the patient may have more than one diagnosis. The ICD-10 system may be preferred over the alternative DSM-IV.

When there is little or ambivalent clinical evidence, making it difficult to produce a firm differential diagnosis, the candidate must make it clear how further information is to be collected within the management plan of the case.

In presenting the case to the examiner, the candidate builds up evidence supporting the diagnosis with which he or she concludes the presentation.

You will also be expected to present an aetiology, and this skill can be practised according to the next exercise.

Group Exercise: Aetiology

Candidates at Part II Clinicals are usually asked to comment on the aetiology of the cases that they present. This can seem straightforward, but there are several ways of thinking about aetiology.

Traditionally candidates talk about precipitating, predisposing and perpetuating factors, but you can also think about the problem in biological, social and psychological terms.

As an awareness exercise gather together a group of colleagues and get them all to set aside an hour or so for the following exercise. A flipchart or whiteboard would be useful.

1   Choose a possible diagnosis for a case that you might encounter in the exam, e.g. depression or anorexia nervosa.
2   One of the group should draw Table 1 on the flipchart or whiteboard.
3   Consider factors that could fit into the nine cells: biological precipitating factors, psychological precipitating factors and so on.
4   As an additional twist to the exercise ask the group to cite research evidence for the factors or perform the same exercise after a specific patient case conference.

Table 1:   Aetiology exercise

	Biological	Psychological	Social
Precipitating			
Predisposing			
Perpetuating			

Constructing the management plan

The management plan is more the preserve of the Part II examination rather than the Part I, which focuses on psychopathology and differential diagnosis. Part I candidates should therefore read the following for interest's sake. The initial part of the management concerns the recruitment of further data to substantiate the diagnosis. The management plan should be divided into two (*see* Box 3).

Box 3   Management plan

			Data collection
	Treatment		
Early management:	Physical		
		Psychological	
		Social	
			Data collection
	Treatment		
Later management:	Physical		
		Psychological	
		Social	

Using headings of this nature, the candidate is less likely to omit important components.

The prognosis

As with management, prognosis is usually explored in the Part II examination only. Any statements you make must be justifiable. The clear-cut case is a relative rarity and to say the prognosis is good, poor or bad without qualification will almost certainly lead to further questioning by the examiner.

The examinee may get away with general terms that do not commit, providing a framework for further discussion within the examination; terms such as 'guarded' or 'cautiously optimistic'. These phrases mean relatively little on their own and might lead to further examination. The best approach is to consider the prognosis in terms of immediate (concerning the particular episode) and longer term. In this context the examinee can present the immediate prognosis as good but draw attention to the poorer long-term prognosis. An example of such a case is a patient presenting with depression who has a history of recurrence or strong personality traits that might make the individual prone to relapse.

Examination time

Time spent with the patient

This is the critical part of the Clinical. How the candidate spends this time determines to a great extent whether the examination is passed or failed.

The objectives are:

- to examine the patient
- to establish a differential diagnosis
- to construct a management plan
- to work out the prognosis
- to rehearse the presentation.

When the examinee first enters the room where the patient is waiting the anxiety will be high but reduces quite quickly. Some examinees will 'freeze' initially. Some suggested ways of overcoming this initial anxiety are listed below.

- Introduce oneself to the patient, explain the exam set-up and that, because time is against you, you may have to cut them short. Try to get the patient 'on your side' as much as possible.
- Take three or four minutes to write out the headings of the presentation (as above), well spaced on a side of paper (a crib sheet). This can be used as a guide during the history taking; it may also be of use later in the examination. This exercise gives the candidate a sense of mastery and will focus thinking, taking the edge off any anxiety. The examinee can now get on with taking the history, taking notes as normal. This should be completed with 10 or 15 minutes to spare at the end for thinking time.

Write down the differential diagnoses. Five broad headings can be considered:

- psychoses (schizophrenias etc.)
- organic
- neuroses (including eating disorders)
- personality
- affective disorders.

It is often useful to have a short classification list in mind as one of the common fears of examinees is that 'something' has been missed. Such a list offers a simple clinical 'sieve'.

The next stage is to write down one-word cues covering the main salient features of the case under each of the headings on the crib sheet (*see* Box 4). This will allow presentation of the case to the examiners without reading from notes word for word.

The last five to 10 minutes of the time left to the candidate can be best spent in presenting the case. This can be done by asking the patient to sit quietly for a few minutes. As the candidate you might turn to face the wall and present the case to yourself in a muttered voice. It is quite important to go through this verbatim as, in doing so, you will not fall into the trap of taking short cuts and will therefore have to think the case through. More importantly, you will be going into the examination having already presented the case.

It may also be worth thinking about likely items the examiners will ask you to demonstrate when you interview the patient in their presence. Key factors of psychopathology may be chosen by the examiners. You could alert the patient beforehand to the kind of questions that you may be asking later. Remember the patient will be just as anxious as you about performing in front of the examiners.

Box 4 An example crib sheet.

Crib sheet summary:

Patient's ID: Mr Pretend, 42 years, engineer, not worked for six months, married, in hospital two weeks (referred by GP)

History of present complaint:
>   Three months ago: saw road traffic accident
>   Cries most days
>   Early morning wakening
>   Diurnal variation
>   Irritable
>   Sex drive down
>   Appetite loss
>   Lack of energy
>   Frightened of being away from wife

Family history: Mother: long-term 'nerve' trouble

Personal history:
>   Father died when patient was six
>   Disturbed elder brother: violent, drugs, theft
>   Difficult schooling: Mum kept him at home
>   Job after school

Lived with Mum until married at 35

Married

Teetotal

No previous psychiatric history

Personality: Dependent, low confidence, prone to withdrawal when under stress

MSE (mental state examination):

Appearance and behaviour: weepy, poor eye contact, stooped, wrings hands, dishevelled

Talk: quiet voice, poor spontaneity, monosyllabic

Mood: sad, low self-esteem

Thought: hopeless, pessimistic, self-depreciative, non-delusional, no suicidal thoughts or plans

Percept. NAD

Cognition: some psychomotor retardation

Differential:

Depression

Dependent traits in personality (NB: early loss)

Management:

Immediate: data collection

Physical: examination, blood tests

Psychiatric: observe for endogenous features, sleep and appetite monitoring, assign key nurse to explore psychology (NB: watch for suicidal ideation)

Social: SW and examine domestic and work dynamic. Explore premorbid personality

Treatment:
- Physical: commence antidepressant
- Psychiatric: key worker to build relationship
- Social: depends on social assessment

Longer term:
- Physical: treat conditions found
- Psychiatric: management of medication; duration and compliance
- Psychosocial: psychotherapy

Prognosis:

Short term: good

Long term: dependent personality will make him vulnerable to future stress. Possible risk of recurrence

Presenting the case

The presentation should begin with a very brief introduction to the case, giving the name, age, occupation and where and with whom he/she lives, and the duration and nature (inpatient/outpatient) of current contact with the psychiatric service. This assessment should fill 10 minutes or so.

Having just spent an hour with the case and having already rehearsed the presentation, the examinee should be confident enough to use the crib sheet. This allows eye contact with the examiners and gets the examinee out of the temptation of reading notes.

The examinee must demonstrate that he/she is confident and organised. Keep good eye contact with the examiners. Reply to questions using the first person.

When psychopathology is referred to in the presentation, a verbatim example is often asked for, so be prepared. It is important that the examinee has the courage of conviction concerning the presence or absence of psychopathology, stating firmly whether the patient is or is not exhibiting the phenomenon.

Do not include diagnoses within the differential that cannot be specifically justified. A great mistake is to be over-inclusive and then to be made a fool of when one cannot explain why it was included, except for 'safety' reasons.

Avoid the term 'organic' in differential diagnoses. If the patient is thought to be suffering from an illness of this nature, then try to be specific and present evidence as to why this diagnosis had been thought of.

When giving the mental state examination, make sure that the appearance of the case is not, for example, just described as 'depressed' but as 'a person with poor eye contact, brimming of the eyes, hunched shoulders, wringing of the hands'. Spend a little time on the appearance and behaviour; describe important features of the personal presentation that contribute towards the differential diagnosis. Such a description is quite impressive.

When the patient is interviewed in front of the examiners be careful to show your awareness of the discomfort that the patient might be experiencing. Turn your chair sideways to the examiner, facing the patient and not the examiners. This makes the interview into a two-way interchange, looks impressive to the examiner and makes the situation much more controllable.

If asked a question by the examiner that is ambiguous or needs clarification, do not hesitate to ask for clarification.

Read and be aware of the guidelines issued by the Royal College on the time generally allocated to items such as 'presentation' and 'patient interview' (*see* Table 2). Please also do the exercises on aetiology and related topics in the rest of the book!

Table 2:   Guide to time spent with examiners in Part II Clinical

Assessment	10 minutes (approx)
Interview with patient	5 minutes (approx)
Management	10 minutes (approx)
Prognosis	10 minutes (approx)
Further discussion	5 minutes (approx)

With practice the candidate will become adept at interviewing the patient, arranging information and will have enough time for a brief rehearsal. The essence of passing the Clinical Examination is to go into it confident and organised. To achieve this it is essential to control anxiety; this is done by extensive rehearsal in the context of a well-established routine which is fail safe.

Some general points

First, the candidates should be assured that examiners do not work to a 'quota system' with a fixed number of passes or fails to allocate. Each candidate is treated on their own merits (or lack of them) and assessed independently by each examiner before a mark is agreed. There is also no way in which performance in the Clinical part of the exam can influence marks in the Patient Management Problems. Each is marked by a separate pair of examiners who are unaware of the candidate's mark in the other section. Examiners are also unaware of any previous exam attempts by the candidate.

Each pair of examiners will usually consist of one general adult psychiatrist and one with a special interest. They are asked to declare any previous knowledge of the candidate before the examination begins (hence the photograph you supply). Despite this a high degree of specialist knowledge is not required; breadth rather than depth is more useful and certainly less irritating.

Although examiners follow a marking scheme the examination process is, by its very nature, a subjective one and is far from an exact science. Candidates can, therefore, help themselves by improving their presentation and discussion skills and should take every opportunity to do so with their consultant and senior training colleagues and peers. Although good technique will probably never allow a poor candidate to pass the exam it can certainly ensure otherwise good candidates do not fail. Practice in history taking, presentation and discussion should be carried out until it becomes second nature to present cases in an orderly, concise and systematic way. This also provides a 'cushion' and prevents panic should something out of the ordinary occur on the big day, e.g. a mute or uncooperative patient. At the end of the exam, whether Clinical or PMP, you should leave the examiners with the impression they have been discussing an interesting case with a courteous, competent and safe colleague with good interpersonal and decision-making skills.

A dozen points to remember

1 Time management is important. Allow plenty of travelling time and, if the exam centre is some distance away, consider an overnight stay close by. Within the exam allow plenty of time to collect your thoughts before the patient leaves you. This time should be spent thinking of aspects of the case which are likely to come up and what you might be asked to demonstrate with the patient present (rehearse this).
2 Try to allocate time to the various components of your presentation. Some cases will lead to detailed discussion of history and mental state with little emphasis on treatment. Other cases have a relatively straight-forward history and discussion will hinge around management and prognosis. The examiners will be aware of this and take it into account in their marking. What you leave out can be just as important as what you include.
3 Always perform some form of risk assessment with reference to self-injurious behaviour or risk to others.
4 Always assess prognosis and perform physical examination as appropriate. These are awarded specific marks and often contribute to failure if not performed adequately.
5 Treatment always has four components: pharmacological, physical, psychological and social. The relative importance of each varies from case to case but each should be considered for potential discussion.
6 Ensure you have detailed knowledge of the role of all members of multidisciplinary teams in assessment and treatment. Do not attempt to amuse the examiner by making 'humorous' disparaging remarks about social workers, clinical psychologists and so on – the examiner may well be having a meaningful relationship with one.

7 Make sure you can discuss the working arrangements for CPA, care in the community and Mental Health Act treatment. Understand the concept and role of 'key worker'.

8 Differential diagnosis should be concise and systematic. Brief reasons for excluding conditions should be given. Remember that common things occur commonly. Examiners are rarely impressed with displays of small islands of erudition in an ocean of ignorance. Know what tests you would request to clarify your diagnosis and how to prioritise them, e.g. full neurological examination before MRI scan.

9 Remember simple things like introducing the patient to the examiners when asked to bring them in. (Remembering the examiners' names always impresses.) You will be marked not only on how you elicit the information required of you but on your handling of the interview and behaviour towards the patient overall.

10 Please listen carefully to the questions the examiners ask you. There will often be a clue in the wording: 'Do you think the patient might be a danger to others?' or 'Would you consider any other treatment?' are usually cues for a positive response. Much valuable time is lost in trying to return candidates to the point if they wander off at a tangent. This is especially important towards the end of the Clinical Examination where the examiners may be trying to fill gaps in the last few minutes and in the PMP exam where conciseness is especially important.

11 Do not waste time in the PMP asking the examiner to clarify the question. The information you are given should be enough to answer if you have listened properly.

12 Finally, don't forget examiners are human and examining is a tiring process. Body language of examiners is a poor guide to your performance: some are twitchy, some still, some are alert, some appear drowsy. Some will tend to interrupt a lot while others are content to let the candidate go on and on ... and on ... and on .... Ability to deal with such behaviours should be regarded as a legitimate clinical and social skill. Do not be put off by this or by the presence of a third examiner. He or she is there to monitor the performance of the examiners and general conduct of the exam by the College and has no influence on the mark you receive.

Group Exercise: Formulation

As an exercise, formulating cases in a formal manner has rather lamentably fallen by the wayside. Although formulation was once considered very much the epitome of psychiatry this once-routine exercise in synthesis is rarely performed except in artificial circumstances such as case conferences and the Membership examination.

As a group, take two cases that someone has worked up to a fairly confident level of detail and work through the scheme in Table 3, listing factors for the headings in each case.

Although the Part I examination does not formally cover management, it is never too early to start watching how others manage cases. The Part I clinical approach is somewhat cross-sectional, but the longitudinal view of a patient and their management is what is required of the Part II candidate and this shift in viewpoint is a crucial one that cannot be made too early. Some aspects of management are timeless, and some are governed by legislation and governmental policy – these change from time to time, but you would be advised to have a shrewd idea as to how the clinical team works and how to reduce risks, using legislation and risk registers where necessary.

Remember too that although it's good to be comprehensive in your formulation, if you mention something in passing it can be explored in detail. For instance, you might aim to be comprehensive in discussing, say, a 16-year-old patient assessed after an overdose. You might justifiably mention doing investigations, and social investigations would be just about mandatory. (What social investigations do you think these would be?) However, if you blithely mentioned doing 'routine' blood tests on a 16-year-old, or 'airily' mentioned psychological tests the examiners would very probably ask which tests and why. Blood screening tests would be unlikely to pick up pathology on a 16-year-old, and you would have to have a clear hypothesis in mind before requesting psychological 'investigations'.

Table 3:   Putting it all together

Differential diagnosis	Aetiology	Investigations	Management
Exclude organic	Biological	Biological	Biological
Psychotic disorders	Social	Social	Social
Neurotic disorders	Psychological	Psychological	Psychological
Personality issues and disorders			
	and/or		*Also consider*
			Clinical team
	Precipitating		Risk management
	Predisposing		Care programme
	Perpetuating		Mental Health Act

MRCPsych Part II: Patient Management Problems

General approach

The Patient Management Problems (PMP) examination lasts for half an hour, during which two examiners pose a variety of problems for you to answer. Candidates are presented with three vignettes and will be marked by two examiners. All candidates sitting the examination at the same date and time will be examined against the same vignettes.

For each vignette candidates are assessed on an 11-point scale ranging from 10 (excellent) to 0 (very poor). A grade of 5 or more is required for a pass in the PMP.

An example of such a PMP from the College website is:

In your outpatient clinic you see a 25-year-old married woman who presents with symptoms of depressed mood and anxiety over a two-year period. Her marriage is under stress. She discloses to you that she was repeatedly abused by her stepfather between the ages of 8 and 12. She has never told anyone about it and insists it is confidential.

The problem is then followed by a general and open-ended questions such as:

How would you assess and manage this situation?

Following this the examiner may use various probes to try and get at their objectives for the question.

The key to the PMP is to appear competent and confident, although not overly so. The examiners must be left with the impression that you would be safe as a consultant. Wild guesses, extraordinary body language, and blatant attempts to show off esoteric knowledge will ruin this impression. As much as anything, examiners are interested in whether you have a strategy for analysing problems, which can be generalised, in your clinical life.

Listen carefully to the problem outlined by the first examiner. The problem should not be over-long or over-detailed. What detail there is in the question is usually vital to the diagnosis or management so try to use all the detail in your reply. Address routine matters first – in assessing patients there are steps which you might take for granted but, unless you mention them, the examiner will have no idea whether you know them or not. The difficulty here is in balancing the need to explain yourself against the distinct possibility of boring the examiners. You alone can judge this in the exam setting. Sometimes examiners will move candidates on to the area they are particularly interested in if they are satisfied that your general approach is correct. Another strategy for the candidate is to 'go for the jugular' and address the most important part of the PMP first.

If the PMP sounds like a 'barn-door' case of neuropsychiatric complications of systemic lupus erythematosus you could say this immediately, but almost in the same breath you must emphasise that you would still go through the usual careful assessment procedure that you always do. This upfront strategy avoids the impression that you are waffling around, talking about assessment, when you haven't a clue as to what the diagnosis might be.

There is no ideal way to answer PMPs that will work with all PMPs for all candidates and all examiners. PMPs can be in diverse subspecialities – learning disability, child psychiatry, forensic psychiatry and others. Your main asset will be the ability to think 'on your feet'. In terms of preparation you should begin practising your skills for the PMP exam as early as possible. Ward rounds and case conferences are good training grounds for voicing your thoughts on patient management. You may also find peer groups useful in practising PMP exam technique. A trio of exam candidates can act in turn as candidates and examiners, having each thought up several PMP-style questions.

During the exam itself the PMPs you are working on may evolve. After you have discussed assessment, the examiners could feed back investigations such as EEG or MRI scan reports. You may have to moderate your initial impressions. After you have formed a working differential diagnosis, the examiners might ask you for your ideal management. Remember that management may include pharmacological, family, social, and individual psychological interventions in a variety of settings (day hospital, outpatients, day centres, community clinics and inpatients). You must be confident to talk about the management of easy and resistant cases of depression and schizophrenia. An increasing emphasis may be placed in the future on knowledge of psychological techniques. How is a behavioural programme structured in detail? What goes into a cognitive-behavioural diary in managing bulimia? If you don't know something in the exam, try to apply basic principles, but don't present dangerous wild guesses, say, about the exact dosage regime of phenelzine.

You will have gained the impression from the above that the PMP exam is very interactive. Both examiners will ask you PMPs and they will have different styles to which you will need to adapt, although their approach is standardised as far as is possible by initial training as examiners and the sometime presence of Royal College observers who may take the form of a 'silent' fourth person in the room.

Some Patient Management Problems will require you to refer to legal procedures used in compulsory admissions for assessment and treatment. The College is aware that, depending on where exam candidates live and work, their familiarity with the English and Welsh Mental Health Act may vary. If you are most familiar with Irish or Scottish legislation, you should make this clear to the examiners in the PMPs and the Clinical test. This will avoid any misunderstanding on the examiners' part. In the following PMPs and responses, we have referred to the 1983 Mental Health Act in use in England and Wales.

The exam may focus on particular difficulties in management, such as how to manage resistant depression or schizophrenia. These and other problems in management that you should be fully conversant with are usefully discussed in:

- Hawton K and Cowen P (1990) *Dilemmas and Difficulties in the Management of Psychiatric Patients*. Oxford University Press, Oxford.

Further hints on PMPs

The first aspect to take into account is *how the examiners see you*. You could show professorial knowledge to your peers, or be praised *ad nauseam* by the consultants you work with, but none of that counts on the day. All that matters is the 30 minutes the examiners see of you. Before turning to consider how you should set about answering their questions, let us first pay attention to the first impressions they will form of you as you walk in the room and sit facing them across the table. First impressions should not be that important, but examiners are human (believe it or not!) so first impressions count for a great deal. Also, if you dress and adopt a posture that looks as if you mean business, then your attitude when answering the questions will tend to follow the same path.

Your appearance should look as if you will be a competent consultant psychiatrist (which, after all, is what the exam is all about). This generally means wearing a dark suit (men) or something equivalent (women). In my (female) opinion, women should wear a skirt (not too short) and if they have long hair, preferably have it neatly tied back. Having said that, the overriding rule should be that you feel comfortable and reasonably natural in whatever you wear: it is no good dressing up to look like someone you are not, as this is likely to make you feel uneasy while talking, and perhaps come across as unconfident to the examiners (more of that later).

Your posture is also crucial. Think about how you will walk into the room and sit down! That may sound daft, but if your head is lifted high and you walk in boldly, perhaps immediately making eye contact with one of the examiners, and then sit down in a calm manner, that will all be to your benefit. Think about your body language while you are sitting. We are all so used to making judgements about patients by the way they sit in a chair, yet are surprised if other psychiatrists do the same to us.

Sit fully on the chair; sitting on the edge will make you look anxious and hence unconfident. You may say that the examiners should realise that any candidate would naturally be feeling anxious, so it should not matter. Unfortunately it does matter. Firstly, the examiners are themselves quite anxious (they may not have met each other before; one of them may not have examined before) so the last thing they want is for someone to sit there and make them feel worse! Secondly, any impression that you are feeling unconfident almost invariably leads to the erroneous impression that you are also incompetent. If there is one thing that you have to convince the examiners of, it is that you are basically a competent and safe psychiatrist. So you should try at all costs not to display your natural anxiety.

Think of yourself going into the exam as a salesperson, selling yourself instead of computers but using the same principles. Make as much eye contact as possible with the examiner who is questioning you (without staring). If you really cannot bear looking straight at the whites of the examiner's eyes, practice looking at a spot on the wall at the examiner's eye level, behind him: this will give the impression that you are looking at him when you are not! Also, don't forget to smile. This will prevent you looking unsure while you are thinking of your answers.

Many salespeople practise their technique either in front of a mirror or in front of a video camera. You must do the same. It really is an exercise worth putting yourself through. I suggest that you find a friend or colleague who can act as a mock examiner (preferably someone doing the exam at the same time as you, so that you can both inflict equal torture on each other). Lay the room out similarly to an exam room: the examiner should sit behind a table, and your chair be directly facing him or her. Place the video camera behind the examiner, focused directly onto the candidate; that way the picture will truly be of you as the examiners see you. Then go through a mock viva. It does not really matter what questions are asked; all that is required is that they put you under some pressure (without deteriorating to an argument!) so that your demeanour and attitude when under stress can be looked at.

Answering the questions posed also requires some practice. There is a convention that your answer should follow the same route as your formulation in the clinical exam would. So you always start with assessment (have a schema in your head of what you run through in a history, mental state, physical examination so that you do not miss anything out); investigation; management. Bear in mind also the triad of 'physical, psychological and social'; and remember that histories can be obtained from individual patients, but also from close relatives, whole families, other agencies (like social workers) or institutions (like employers or schools), as well as from previous case notes!

In medicine there is often an exception to an 'always'. I would say that the exception to your answer 'always' beginning with assessment is if there is some information of overriding importance that you want to make sure you have time to let the examiner know you know. This generally arises in situations where life is somehow in danger. For example, if given a description of someone who is or could be suicidal, I would begin with: 'My prime concern here is for the patient's safety, and I am concerned that she may be a suicide risk, but I would begin by assessing...'. This shows the examiners you are thinking safely, but allows you also to then go through the conventional pattern of answering, and you can return to discuss the suicidal intent in more detail later on.

The exception described above should not be abused. There is often a temptation, especially when adrenalin is pumping through your veins, to envisage some rare small-print syndrome that might fit the description given by the examiners. By all means keep that whim at the back of your mind, to earn extra points after you have given your textbook reply, but stop yourself from mentioning it before anything else. Common things occur commonly, and the examiners will be perfectly satisfied if you have a good working knowledge of the main syndromes.

If you are asked a question you do not understand, do not waste time, just ask the examiner to repeat it; the chances are the other examiner had not understood it either. Do not be thrown by questions about the obscure: everybody has their own ceiling, and it may just be that they are testing you to see how well you can perform.

When the examiner goes on to the next PMP, try to put the previous one completely out of your head. You have to earn points on each one, so try to begin with a completely clean slate each time.

Below is a selection of PMPs by different authors. They are followed by sample answers. The responses are not meant as ideal or 'model' answers, only as examples of possible ways of answering the PMP. You might like to try to formulate your own answers before reading our examples. There is some representation of how interactive the PMPs can be because, in our examples, the examiners do come back with supplementary questions or probes. In practice there is likely to be more interaction.

Sample PMPs

1 The asthmatic

The medical team asks you to see a 21-year-old girl who is currently on a medical ward for a severe attack of asthma. She may soon need ventilation. The patient is refusing this and wants to take her own discharge. Her asthma is usually controlled with inhalers but she stopped these herself. Her asthma is complicated by a small pneumothorax. She has seen a psychiatrist in the past. She has a history of deliberate self-harm dating from the age of 14.

On interview, she is breathless, and has successfully detached herself from a drip of hydrocortisone. She has also been treated with nebulised bronchodilators. She gives a history of low mood with an onset six weeks before the asthma attack, and describes current tearfulness, poor appetite, and early morning wakening. She has ideas of worthlessness, delusions of guilt and second-person auditory hallucinations telling her that she should kill herself. The patient is disorientated in time, but not in place or person.

How would you respond to the physicians' request for help?

This is a complex case, which would need careful assessment, but also seems to merit a swift response. On what I have been told there are grounds for using the Mental Health Act to detain this patient. Firstly there is evidence of a mental disorder (low mood preceding the attacks and current psychotic features) and, secondly, the patient is at risk of harming herself because of self-hate and second-person auditory hallucinations telling her to kill herself. It may also be that her decision to reject treatment is based on a desire to harm herself. On this basis there would be a case for not allowing her to discharge herself and using a Section. Since she is an inpatient, Section 5.2 *could* be applied by the RMO (Responsible Medical Officer), but Section 2 proceedings might be preferable. This would allow treatment of her mental disorder, but treatment for any physical illness would fall under Common Law. Her mental disorder affects her ability to give valid consent at this time (given that there are psychotic features and disorientation). After a Section has been invoked, joint evaluation and treatment by medical and psychiatric teams would be necessary. Their aims would be to improve her respiratory function and assess and treat her mental disorder.

There is a history of low mood preceding the asthma attack, which might indicate an underlying depressive illness, although she is quite young to develop this. I would take a careful drug history. For instance, had she been on steroids for any great length of time? Steroids could have produced her psychotic state. Her disorientation could be due to hypoxia. As her respiratory function improved, her disorientation might improve, and so might some of her psychotic symptoms.

At this point the examiner intervenes to give further information. Some second-person auditory hallucinations had preceded the asthma attack, and continued after her asthma attack was over. She was not on steroids before this admission.

In this case a major depressive episode seems more likely, with a hypoxic disorientation overlying this. The patient or an informant could give a clear history of the depressive illness.

So, given that she is now on the Mental Health Act Section 2, how would you treat her?

This would have to be in conjunction with the physicians, but I would be keen to gain rapid control of her depressive illness. ECT might be the treatment of choice, if there were no respiratory contraindications. Her respiratory function and recent pneumothorax might concern the anaesthetist. An antidepressant like fluoxetine or sertraline might be an alternative. If there were associated behavioural disturbance, I would recommend a neuroleptic with less sedative properties like haloperidol.

Have you any thoughts about her personality, given her history of deliberate self-harm? She has cut her wrists in the past and taken overdoses as a teenager.

My assessment would also include her account and an informant's account of her pre-morbid personality. I would consider the possibility that there was a personality disorder. Her asthma attack (precipitated by a failure to take treatment) might have been a deliberate act of self-harm too. However, given the immediate presentation, I would be careful to assess and treat any depressive illness.

Further reading

- Jourdan JB and Glickman L (1991) Reasons for requests for evaluation of competency in a municipal general hospital. *Psychosomatics*. **32**: 413–16.
- Kopelman LM (1990) On the evaluative nature of competency and capacity judgements. *Int J Law Psychiatr*. **13**: 309–29.
- Wear AN and Brahams D (1991) To treat or not to treat: the legal, ethical and therapeutic implications of treatment refusal. *J Med Ethics*. **17**: 131–5.

BG

2 A panic attack

A casualty SHO asks you to see a 45-year-old lady. She has just had a 'panic attack' and fainted while shopping in the centre of town. She talks to you of her anxieties about her daughter's impending wedding (she had been in town to buy a hat for the wedding). You notice that she smells of alcohol, which she spontaneously explains. A shopkeeper had given her some brandy to revive her. However, on physical examination you notice that she has palmar erythema, a tremor and a pulse rate of 104 beats per minute.

How would you propose to further assess and manage her?

The smell of alcohol and the palmar erythema would make me suspicious that this lady abuses alcohol. I would review her alcohol history particularly carefully, seeking confirmation from a relative or other informant. The informant might be able to give valuable information about the panic attack, which I am unclear about. Was this really a panic attack induced by general anxieties about a forthcoming wedding? Or was it perhaps a symptom of agoraphobia, or an attack of syncope, or an alcohol withdrawal fit? The history would clarify some of these issues, particularly about the form of the actual attack itself. It would be important to exclude medical causes such as a rhythm disturbance.

An examiner intervenes to inform the candidate that there was no irregularity in the pulse, but that there was tachycardia.

Yes, so I would be interested not only in the history and physical examination but also in some investigations. Specifically, I would request an ECG, but also a full blood count (in case of anaemia), a urea and electrolytes (for dehydration) and serum glucose (to exclude hyper- or hypoglycaemia). A thyroid function test (TFT) would be important to exclude hyperthyroidism which might be the cause of any anxiety and tachycardia. Liver function tests (LFTs) including a gamma-GT and the MCV (mean corpuscular volume) on her full blood count might exclude prolonged alcohol abuse.

Let us suppose that all the initial casualty investigations come back normal. Perhaps her tachycardia resolves when she has talked to you a bit more about her difficulties at home. You have been careful enough to get the medium-term investigations like LFTs and TFTs done and, obviously, are awaiting their results.

Well then I would be interested in her past psychiatric history. Were there any episodes of agoraphobia in the past? Has her GP given her any treatment for anxiety? Perhaps with benzodiazepines? And particularly ask about her family relationships. Perhaps the panic is to do with her daughter leaving home, some structural change in the family. I would try to get an opportunity to talk to the husband...

> *The examiner interrupts because he is satisfied with this line of enquiry and has only a few points to cover before closing down. He acknowledges the role that psychological factors may play in the presentation, but asks what pharmacological alternatives there would be to psychotherapeutic measures.*

Particularly if there was an element of general low mood, an antidepressant such as paroxetine or imipramine might help. Both have been reported to be of value in panic disorders. MAOIs have been used for agoraphobia and panic disorder, but there might be difficulties using irreversible MAOIs in someone with an alcohol problem. So I would perhaps consider an MAOI such as moclobemide which does not have such severe dietary restrictions as the older irreversible MAOIs. Propranolol *could* have a role if there were a more generalised anxiety, but you would have to check whether there was any predisposition to asthma. Benzodiazepines would certainly reduce the anxiety, but would not be of any medium- or long-term benefit.

BG

3 The school non-attender

> *A school medical officer sends you a referral, a 13-year-old girl who has barely attended school in the last half-term (it is now halfway through the Autumn term). She has always been a good attendee until now. Her schoolwork has also suffered. She was a most able pupil. Now she has slipped to being near the bottom of the class.*
>
> *How would you set about managing this problem?*

This case requires outpatient assessment, but does need a swift response as her schoolwork has apparently suffered quite markedly. The assessment will involve seeing the girl herself and making a family assessment. I would get information (if parents allow) from the school and any other interested parties such as the Educational Welfare Officer.

A very important area to cover in the history of the presenting problem is whether or not this is school refusal or truancy. Is she staying at home with her parents' knowledge? Or is she pretending to them that she is attending, and either not turning up at all, or leaving very early in the school day? Does she truant in a group with friends, or (more worryingly) on her own? If she is truanting, what does she do during the day? (Drug abuse, glue-sniffing or shoplifting are particular worries.)

A clear indication of the duration of the problem is required – did it really start after the end of the summer holidays? What were the antecedents? Is she currently attending school? What statutory moves have been made to get her back to school? An indication of whether the school has a sympathetic attitude towards her case or not is useful.

> *The examiner explains further that this is a case of truancy. Occasionally she truants with other girls (who were not previously her friends). However, much of the time she never turns up at school, and appears to go into town on her own. She denies any substance abuse and simply says she wanders round the shops all day. The school has been so worried about her behaving out of character that no legal moves have yet been made.*
>
> *Her mother says that she became more moody, and more difficult to talk to, since her periods began. Her periods started just after the end of the previous summer term.*
>
> *What does this make you think of?*

Of prime importance here is this girl's probable very low mood. I would elicit any suicidal ideas or plans. Evidence we already have for a depression would be her truanting alone, deteriorating school performance, and a change in behaviour at home as well.

My next concern would be the cause of this depression. The timing of the problems just after the menarche is vital. There are several ways in which the onset of periods can be disruptive for a teenager. The impact may depend upon what the girl expected beforehand and how her family (and especially mother) reacted to her menarche. Her peers may have teased her about it. There is also the possibility of sexual abuse and its consequences.

4 The soiler

> *A GP asks you to see a six-year-old boy who soils himself at least once every day. How would you set about this?*

I would obtain a thorough history. It would be worth finding out from the GP what investigations and treatment(s) have been attempted, and over what length of time. The whole family should be seen, to take a history, including duration and onset of the problem, also the precise circumstances around current episodes of soiling. It is very important to determine whether the boy has been adequately toilet trained. A clear past history, including his position in the family, and current family and school circumstances, is required. This assessment may need several meetings with the family. Teachers' opinions and reports should be sought.

The pattern of the soiling itself will need examining. Is aggression a main motive behind it? Are there associated behaviours such as smearing? Is he constipated (suggesting a more retentive pattern)? Eliciting the precise antecedents and consequences of specific incidents of soiling can be very informative.

The examiner elaborates the history by explaining that the soiling only occurs at home, never at school, and follows a retentive pattern. He was clean and dry from the age of two until six months ago. Furthermore, his parents separated over a year ago, and are getting a divorce. The boy is the elder of two children, his sister being four years old and showing no problems at all.

What else do you want to know?

The parents' separation and divorce seem linked in time to the start of the symptoms. I would ask about the state of the parents' marriage beforehand, and also about current difficulties. I would like to know precisely what the boy has been told about what is going on.

The father is a long-distance lorry driver who used to be away in Europe for several days at a time. He left his wife a year ago for another woman (who was expecting a baby by him, which was born six months ago). Both his original children stayed with their mother. The mother had been very upset by the break-up. Since then, her husband had started requesting access, but even before that they were frequently rowing about this.

How would you now manage this case?

The access dispute is the major perpetuating factor here, so resolution of this between the parents will be a major help in relieving the stress borne by the boy. Conciliation work may be required for this.

The divorce may not have been adequately explained to the six-year-old, so it should be ensured that the situation is clearly and unambiguously explained to him. Ideally, both parents should do this together: but this may not be practicable, so they may need to do this independently.

Addressing these two issues will be tackling the probable causes of the encopresis. However, his soiling may have taken on the nature of a habit, so that, even when these factors have been removed, behavioural techniques may also be required, including star charts, consistent reactions to soiling, and positive rewards (specific to the child himself) for remaining clean. A hierarchy of achievable targets should be created. Also, the boy may be so severely constipated at presentation as to require 'clearing out' with laxatives or even, in exceptional circumstances, an enema before the behavioural treatment programme can be embarked on.

5 The addict

A 26-year-old woman is referred to your drug dependency clinic by a consultant obstetrician. She is 12 weeks pregnant, wants to keep the baby, and has told the obstetrician that she is a heroin addict. How would you proceed?

In order to manage this patient, I would want more information from the patient and an informant. I would want to confirm that she is in fact a heroin addict. I would want to know more about her drug use, her general circumstances, her motivation to stop taking drugs and her knowledge of the health risks she is taking. I would want to be able to discuss other details with the obstetrician.

The first thing is to get a full history of her drug habit. I would want to know which substances, including alcohol, she takes, how much of them, and for how long she has been using them. I would need to know whether she injects now or in the past, and whether she has ever shared needles. Is her habit funded out of legitimate income or crime? If she is a prostitute or has shared needles, there is a risk of hepatitis and HIV. I would ask about any periods of abstinence from drugs or drink and how they were achieved. Has she ever had treatment or help for substance misuse in the past?

I would need to know about her general social circumstances: housing, employment and support from family, friends and/or partner. I would look for any evidence of mental illness, and predisposing, precipitating and maintaining factors for her heroin addiction.

Physical examination would be important for evidence of drug use such as weight loss, constricted pupils, and intravenous puncture marks, venous thromboses, abscesses, sinuses – looking in the groins, neck and legs as well as the arms. Breast veins are sometimes used in late pregnancy. I would also look for any signs of septicaemia or endocarditis. I would take a full blood count, liver function tests, hepatitis and syphilis screening, and might consider offering HIV tests if appropriate. Such testing would need to be after appropriate counselling. Urine samples should be sent on more than one clinic attendance to confirm the presence of opiates (bearing in mind any prescribed medication she might be taking as some of these may interact with testing).

I would assess her motivation to stop taking heroin. Ultimately, she may want to stop completely or become stabilised on oral methadone.

I would, with her permission, interview an informant, perhaps a partner, to check the information I have been given and to enlist their support in her treatment. Discussion of the management with her GP and obstetrician would help.

Since she is in the early stages of pregnancy, she should be stabilised on methadone rather than withdrawing her completely, because of the risk of spontaneous abortion. The methadone could be prescribed mg for mg with heroin, but the starting dose would have to be calculated with great care since the purity of street heroin varies enormously. The first goal would therefore be for her to stop using street heroin, and to stop injecting and any relevant criminal activity.

I mentioned the risks of stopping opiates completely in the first trimester and, for the same reason, reducing her methadone in the first trimester would not be advisable. Reducing her methadone in the last trimester might induce premature labour. It *might* be possible though to reduce her methadone gradually in the middle trimester.

What about any legal implications of her seeking help from you?

At the first appointment, I would have to tell her that I was legally obliged to notify her name to the Chief Medical Officer because there is a register of addicts.

And what about the baby? Would there be any short-term or long-term consequences?

If the patient does not stop taking drugs during pregnancy, the baby is likely to be born drug dependent and would need very careful management of withdrawal symptoms. In the long term, there would be implications if the mother is HIV-positive and if the baby is born HIV-positive. The child would then be at risk in terms of cognitive decline in infancy and HIV-dementia. If there is no HIV infection then the child may still be at risk of conduct or other childhood psychological disorders if their environment is chaotic. There is evidence to suggest that, if the mother continues to use heroin in the years to come, then her child is more likely to use heroin too.

Further reading

- Glynn TJ (1981) From family to peer: a review of transitions of influence among drug using youth. *J Youth Adol.* **10**: 363–83.
- Hepburn M (1993) Drug use in pregnancy. *Br J Hosp Med.* **49**: 1.
- Nurco DN, Hanlon TE and Kinlock TW (1991) Recent research on the relationship between illicit drug use and crime. *Behav Sci Law.* **9**: 221–42.

- Smart RG and Fejer D (1972) Relationships between parental and adolescent drug use. In: W Keup (ed.) *Drug Abuse: current concepts and research*. Charles C Thomas, Illinois.

6 Adolescent depression

A 15-year-old boy is referred to you because of a three-month history of low mood, irritability, anxiety, disturbed sleep and weight loss. He is about to sit his exams and his parents have high expectation for his results. He is finding it difficult to concentrate and to work at his normal standard.

Discuss the child's assessment.

A   Assessment of family, child on own and information from school (with consent).

   - Need to engage with boy and family.
   - History, examination and mental state examination.
   - Aim is to establish a diagnosis, aetiology, severity and protective factors.

B   Risk assessment including suicidal ideas.

C   Likely diagnosis is a depressive disorder; also consider substance misuse. Mention these first before a wider differential diagnosis.

Scenario continues:

You confirm a diagnosis of depressive disorder. The boy is due to sit his exams in four weeks and the family are asking for treatment that will help by then.

Discuss the child's treatment.

A   Advice with regard to the options in the short-term 'bio-psychosocial' perspective needed. This may include writing (after appropriate discussion/consent) to school to allow more time in the exams or focusing on a smaller number of subjects. The relevant exam board may make allowances and base the results on the coursework already submitted. Helping to manage the parents' expectation of the exam results may relieve some of the stress.

B   Formal psychological intervention is likely to be needed but unlikely to resolve all the difficulties in the timescale wanted by the family. CBT has the best evidence base. Some simple anxiety management techniques may be helpful in the short term.

C   Medication may be indicated but caution is needed. Most SSRIs are not now recommended in young people, because of an increase in suicidal ideation (but not completed suicide). Fluoxetine would be the medication with the most favourable side-effect profile. Timescale may be too short in relation to the exams and there is the potential for side effects.

Further reading

- Barrett PM and Ollendick TH (2004) *Handbook of Interventions That Work With Children and Adolescents*. Wiley, Chichester.
- Carr A (2002) *Depression and Attempted Suicide in Adolescence*. PACT2 series. BPS Blackwell, Oxford.
- Federal Drug Administration (FDA) (2004).
- Medicines and Healthcare Products Regulatory Agency (MHRA) (2004).

7 The arsonist

How would you assess a patient referred because of setting a fire?

A key point of the assessment would be of the *patient's dangerousness*. I would take a detailed history of the fire-setting to see if the act was premeditated or impulsive, carried out alone or with others and whether it was part of a pattern of previous fire-setting behaviour. I would be interested in the factors that motivated the patient – such as covering up some other crime, insurance fraud, revenge, political motivation, sexual gratification or re-inforcement, delusional ideation, suicidal ideation, or the wish to appear a hero, perhaps by calling the fire brigade.

I would take a full psychiatric history and make a thorough mental state assessment, looking for evidence of mental illness, mental retardation, alcohol dependence or personality disorder, all of which have been linked to fire-setting behaviour.

An informant would be essential for a corroborative history.

Three groups of arsonist have been described: motivated arsonists – ones motivated by political or financial reward; pathological arsonists suffering from mental illness such as depression, mania, schizophrenia, mental retardation or alcoholism; and a third group who derive sexual enjoyment from fire-setting or who derive better self-esteem from heroic acts at 'their' fire.

What would make you think they were likely to repeat the fire-setting behaviour in the future?

Place on a Supervision Register, previous contact with forensic psychiatry services, history of previous arson, mental retardation and poor insight, dissocial personality disorder, social isolation, and fire-setting reinforced by sexual arousal and masturbation, or reinforced by tension relief.

Further reading

- Gunn J and Taylor PJ (1993) *Forensic Psychiatry – clinical, legal and ethical issues.* Butterworth Heinemann, London, pp.587–98.
- Kolko DJ and Kadzin AE (1991) Motives of childhood firesetters: firesetting characteristics and psychological correlates. *J Child Psychol Psychiatr.* **32**: 535–50.

8 A domiciliary visit

You have been asked to do a domiciliary visit on a 70-year-old woman who lives in a council flat. Her social worker is concerned about self-neglect and her mental state. On arriving at her flat with the social worker the woman speaks to you from her front door but doesn't let you in. She says that she is well and doesn't need to see a doctor. She appears grossly neglected and the flat appears cold, dark, damp and not fit for habitation. She says she hears voices from across the road that say that 'we will get you one day'. She then shuts the door asking you to go away.
   What is the differential diagnosis?

Given the limited information available diagnoses of a paranoid state would include schizophrenia, schizo-affective disorder, mania, depressive disorder, delusional disorder, dementia, delirium and other organic brain disorder (F06).

   How would you proceed from here?

One would have to get corroborative history from various agencies before proceeding. This may include the family, GP, neighbours, social services, mental health services in the region, housing associations and possibly emergency services. Further attempts to see her may result in more success. If this remains unsuccessful it may be worthwhile asking the community mental health nurse to try and make contact with her with or without help of family or neighbours.

   She is subsequently formally admitted to hospital for an assessment. What investigations would you carry out?

A complete physical examination must be done. Investigations should include blood count, urea and electrolytes, full biochemical profile, glucose, urine analysis, B12 and folate, chest X-ray and ECG.

   What other assessments are important?

Assessments from nurses and occupational therapists would be part of the assessment, observing attention to personal care, ability to perform activities of daily living, motivation, social interaction, evidence of psychotic symptoms, diet, sleep pattern and weight. Cognitive assessments including Mini Mental State Examination scores may be helpful.

What may be the indications for neuroimaging in this case?

If there is evidence of cognitive deficits or there are neurological signs on physical examination, neuroimaging techniques such as CT or MRI brain scanning should be considered.

How would you distinguish late-onset schizophrenia disorder from depression in old age presenting with paranoid ideas?

Normal affect, first-rank symptoms of schizophrenia, social isolation and premorbid schizoid or paranoid traits would favour a diagnosis of late-onset schizophrenia. Depressed mood, mood-congruent psychotic symptoms, suicidal thoughts and a past history of mood disorder would favour depression. The time relationship between mood and psychotic symptoms would be an indicator as depressive symptoms usually precede psychotic symptoms in mood disorder. Depression with psychosis is normally accompanied by marked biological symptoms of depression, retardation and neglect.

Further reading

- Anderson N and Jacques A (2004) *Companion to Psychiatric Studies* (7e). Churchill Livingstone, Edinburgh, Chapter 26.

9 Adolescent eating disorder

You are asked to see a 17-year-old girl on a gastroenterology ward. She had been investigated for weight loss but no organic cause was found.
In spite of being given 2500 calories a day for the two weeks of her admission she has not gained weight. Apart from the report of a little diarrhoea, which she attributed to irritable bowel, she has no complaints. She is adamant she is eating her diet. She is a helpful patient, always offering to help the nurses with drinks and meals for the other patients. She is 5' 6" tall and weighs five stone.
What else would you like to know?

The pattern of her weight loss, was she overweight before, normal weight, speed of weight loss, did she go on a diet, what was she eating before, when was her last period, did she exercise, did she binge, vomit, take laxatives, shoplift or steal food, stop eating in front of the family, become reclusive and irritable?

Did she have calluses on her fingers, swollen parotid glands, lanugo hair, thinning of her hair, hypothermia, bradycardia?

Does she like her body; does she think she's thin; does she want to gain weight? Does she spend hours checking her body in front of the mirror?

Is she depressed, obsessive, anxious?

> *Her mother reported that 'A' became vegetarian and started 'healthy eating' which meant she had cut crisps, chocolate and other fattening foods out of her diet. She had never been overweight but her friends at school all went on diets so she thought she should too. When the family said she had lost too much weight she became hostile and stopped eating with them, reporting that she was eating in her room. She was working very hard for her AS levels and achieving very good grades. She had lost weight progressively more rapidly, her periods stopped five months ago and the GP referred her to gynaecology who found no abnormality other than low hormone levels and so referred her to gastroenterology. There was no evidence of an organic cause. She denied binging, vomiting or using laxatives. She had very thin hair, lanugo on her body and had developed mild ankle swelling in hospital.*
>
> *She had rituals about where her possessions were put on the ward and she spent a lot of time in the bathroom. The staff were unclear why.*
>
> *What are your thoughts?*

Does she have an eating disorder? Anorexia nervosa?

Need to work out her body mass index (BMI). Is this less than 17.6? Specialist eating disorder service is required. If rapid weight loss or BMI less than 13.5 this needs consideration for admission to specialist unit where physical monitoring and psychological therapies can be offered.

Age of patient? As she is under 18, may need family therapy and individual therapy.

Is this restrictive or purging subtype? Does she purge? Is her biochemistry normal? Low potassium and sometimes low sodium are associated with severe purging.

Metabolic alkalosis and low serum magnesium need to be corrected before potassium treatment is effective. If mild and the purging stops then dietary changes may suffice. In severe cases potassium supplements are crucial and in emergencies an infusion may be necessary.

Low protein is usually associated with laxative abuse or vomiting.

Mental state: Examine her mental state for mood change, obsessive-compulsive symptoms and eating disorder pathology, i.e. body dissatisfaction, body distortion, body checking. Fear of energy dense foods. Fear of weight gain.

Does she have comorbid depression or OCD?

Is this part of the starvation syndrome or a condition in its own right?

Treatment:

- Save life: re-feeding is crucial.
- Correct physical abnormalities.
- Deal with underlying causes.
- Alter eating disorder distorted thinking.
- Manage life skills.

Don't forget the 20% mortality from this condition.

Further reading

- Brownell K and Fairburn C (1995) *Eating Disorders and Obesity: a comprehensive handbook*. Guilford Press, New York.
- Cooper PJ (1995) *Bulimia Nervosa and Binge Eating: a self help guide using CBT*. Robinson, London.
- Crisp AH (1995) *Anorexia Nervosa: Let Me Be*. Psychology Press, Hove.
- Crisp A and McClelland L (1996) *Anorexia Nervosa: guidelines for assessment and treatment in primary and secondary care*. Psychology Press, Hove.
- Freeman C (2002) *Overcoming Anorexia Nervosa*. Constable Robinson, London.
- Garner D and Garfinkel P (1985) *Handbook of Psychotherapy for Anorexia Nervosa and Bulimia*. Guilford Press, New York.
- Gomez J (1995) *How to Cope With Bulimia*. Sheldon Press, London.
- *International Journal of Eating Disorders* (2005) Vol. 37, Supplement. Special issue on anorexia nervosa. Wiley Publishers.
- *Medical Complications of Eating Disorders*.
- NICE guidelines.
- *Overcoming Bulimia Nervosa and Binge Eating*.
- Schmidt U, Treasure J and Treasure T (1993) *Getting Better Bit(e) by Bit(e): a survival kit for sufferers of bulimia and binge eating disorders*. Psychology Press, London.
- Treasure J (1997) *Anorexia Nervosa: a survival guide for families; friends and sufferers*. Psychology Press, Hove.

KC

10 Advance directives

A patient is admitted informally under your care. The diagnosis is of mania. This is the patient's second episode. The first was some 10 years ago. The patient is at first compliant with medication (lithium and olanzapine). This, however, fails to stop a deterioration in his condition. He becomes increasingly bizarre, hostile and sexually disinhibited. On one occasion there is suspicion that he has touched a female patient in an inappropriate and sexual manner. The situation worsens and the patient is becoming exhausted and dehydrated due to constant activity and a refusal to sit down to eat or drink.

What will you do? Despite optimising meds the condition fails to be brought under control.

The diagnosis should be reviewed. Is compliance really certain? Rapid tranquillisation may be considered with benzodiazepines and antipsychotics. If this fails other options may include ECT.

The patient refuses to consider ECT, saying that he had it 10 years previously and that not only had it failed to work, but that it had caused him to have a CVA [cerebrovascular accident]. You suspect that neither of these facts is true. What other options do you have?

I would speak to his relatives. They may recall whether he ever had ECT and whether it helped or not. They may be sympathetic and may be able to reason with the patient.

His relatives say that the patient did very well on ECT 10 years before but has said, on at least one occasion since then, that if he were ever to be ill again he would not want ECT, irrespective of the consequences. Does that constitute an advance directive and, if so, do you abide by it?

Technically no, because the directive would need to fulfil certain criteria that mere verbal recall of past conversations at some unspecified time in the past would not meet.

An advance directive where treatment is refused would have legal effect provided the person is an adult and medically competent when they made the advance refusal; and the person had the appropriate information to decide this at the time it was made; and the person knew the consequences of the refusal at the time it was made; and the person intended the refusal to apply in the current circumstances; and the person was not acting under the influence of others when they made the decision; and the refusal has not been revoked, nor has the person's conduct (whether by words or actions) been inconsistent with the directive; *and* the person is now mentally incapable of making the decision. If the patient retains capacity, then it is the assessment made at the time which counts.

If you decide to accept that it is a valid advance directive, could you section the patient in order to give ECT?

An advance directive cannot overrule a compulsory treatment decision made if a patient is detained under the Mental Health Act. (Nevertheless, the patient's wishes should always be taken into account whenever any treatment decision is made.)

LF

Index